"*Understanding a Child the Occupational Therapy Way* is compelling and innovative in its focus on celebrating each child and how they experience the world, learn, and behave. Sabrina Adair has written a unique resource for students and parents, explaining complex concepts about development and occupational therapy clearly. She shares cogent stories to illustrate how the interrelationships between a child, their activities, and their environment shape their participation in daily life. Building on solid conceptual frameworks, the book illustrates state-of-the-art strategies to utilize a child's strengths to facilitate change and help them reach their potential."

—**Mary Law, OC, PhD**, *Professor Emerita, McMaster University*

"This is a fabulous book for parents and other caregivers. Warm, wise, and compassionate, this book equips parents with in-depth knowledge and essential insights that help them better understand and help their often complex and always wonderful children using the proven holistic and loving approach that the most effective occupational therapists use to help their young clients and families flourish and thrive."

—**Lindsey Biel, OTR/L**, *Occupational Therapist; co-author*, Raising a Sensory Smart Child; *author*, Sensory Processing Challenges: Effective Clinical Work with Kids and Teens

"As a parent to two young children with diverse and varying needs, I found this book to be a very helpful, informative, and enlightening read. It helped me to shift my focus from the challenge or difficult behavior my child might be exhibiting, to the root cause, and how I can best support my child. It encourages us as parents to ask more questions before we react. This book has helped me to look at my children as whole, complete people, and to guide and clarify my own role as their parent."

—**Pippa Elliott**, *mom of two children ages 4 and 6*

"Tired of fragmented approaches? Sabrina empowers families and professionals to see the whole and foster a shared vision. Her practical section on collaborating ensures everyone, including the child, is working together in the child's best interest. Families and professionals will be excited to delve in and find what works for each unique child and their unique situation. With a shared understanding and vision, we can work together to 'understand a child—to create a world where they belong.'"

—**Hilary Diouf, BA Social Studies**, *Certified Positive Discipline Trainer*

Understanding a Child the Occupational Therapy Way

This book uses an occupational therapy way of thinking to guide the reader towards observing, understanding, and communicating the needs of children to foster a supportive environment.

Presented in accessible, everyday language, this book takes a holistic approach of looking at a child from what makes them a unique person, what activities they are trying to accomplish, and what environment they are in. Each chapter helps readers identify, describe, and clearly articulate a different aspect of the child's environment and how it may affect them, the way that they process different sensory inputs, what their behaviors may be telling us, and how they learn. By recognizing each child's unique story and effectively communicating their story to others, the reader can identify the most effective ways to support a child to meet a child's needs and set them up for success.

Therapists, educators, parents, and childcare workers will all benefit from the simple strategies outlined in this book to enrich a child's learning.

Sabrina E. Adair, MScOT, is a practicing occupational therapist, a mom to four unique and beautiful children, and a passionate advocate for parent empowerment.

Understanding a Child the Occupational Therapy Way

Recognizing and Communicating the Unique Potential of a Child

Sabrina E. Adair

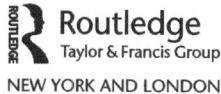

Routledge
Taylor & Francis Group

NEW YORK AND LONDON

First published 2022
by Routledge
605 Third Avenue, New York, NY 10158

and by Routledge
2 Park Square, Milton Park, Abingdon, Oxon, OX14 4RN

*Routledge is an imprint of the Taylor & Francis Group, an informa
business*

Library of Congress Cataloging-in-Publication Data
Names: Adair, Sabrina E., author.
Title: Understanding a child the occupational therapy way :
   recognizing and communicating the unique potential of a child /
   Sabrina E. Adair.
Description: New York, NY : Routledge, 2022. | Includes
   bibliographical references and index.
Identifiers: LCCN 2021013769 (print) | LCCN 2021013770 (ebook) |
   ISBN 9780367763220 (hardback) | ISBN 9780367763206
   (paperback) | ISBN 9781003166405 (ebook)
Subjects: LCSH: Occupational therapy for children.
Classification: LCC RJ53.O25 A33 2022 (print) | LCC RJ53.O25
   (ebook) | DDC 615.8/515083—dc23
LC record available at https://lccn.loc.gov/2021013769
LC ebook record available at https://lccn.loc.gov/2021013770

ISBN: 978-0-367-76322-0 (hbk)
ISBN: 978-0-367-76320-6 (pbk)
ISBN: 978-1-003-16640-5 (ebk)

DOI: 10.4324/9781003166405

Typeset in Times New Roman
by Apex CoVantage, LLC

To Austin, Katelyn, Logan, and Abigail,

I hope the world always recognizes you for your beauty within.

You are capable of amazing things.

Contents

Preface

The feeling of being inadequate as a parent really impacted me when my children were in grade school. Judged by teachers for how your child was reacting or behaving at school. Being questioned by other parents for your child's choices or actions, feeling guilty for not being able to control their behavior. Realizing firsthand what it feels like to have a child who is misunderstood. This is when it really sunk in. We need to remember that our children are not us. Nor can we control who they are or who they will become. They are their own person. There is a belief that we should be able to control everything about them, but it isn't true. Instead, we should seek to understand, support, celebrate, and encourage their uniqueness.

Even as an occupational therapist working with children, I understood then more than ever before how parents or caregivers may feel. It was almost a sense of helplessness. As parents, we are on the same path of discovery as everyone else, working with children to figure out who these children are and what makes them unique. No two children are the same, and no two adults the same. They each have their own unique story. It is a story that needs to be shared.

What I became passionate about was uncovering a child's story so that we could share it with others. I wanted to empower others to really spend the time understanding who these amazing children are. When we could share what makes each child unique, the perspective of those around the child changed. It went from a sense of criticism to a sense of curiosity. Sharing the child's story gave parents, caregivers, teachers, and support workers an understanding of why actions were happening, and they were able to learn how to be proactive in helping a child find their place in the world and belong for who they are.

It wasn't a complicated approach; it was quite simple. I went back to my first occupational therapy class on models and theories and then back to the basics. I was able to answer these two questions:

> *What makes a person who they are?*
> *What will influence a child?*

First, the belief is that a human being is comprised of many characteristics that make them who they are. This is affected by the tasks and activities we are required to accomplish throughout our day, and lastly, these tasks will take place in unique environments that can influence the outcomes. All of these layers will impact one another in some way.

I wrote this book as an encouragement to others who work with children or have children. It is based on the perspective that we need to start from the beginning to understand the whole child and get a sense of what makes them who they are. Sometimes, we get caught jumping to a conclusion before we even know the plot. We can get ahead of ourselves by focusing only on one area of a child's life. We react before we even know the whole story. This book is about taking that step back and keeping our eyes open to look at all aspects of a child. When you have all the information and you know the story, you can delve deeper into the different areas.

As you go through this book, I also encourage you to think about your own life and story. I have included questions in each chapter that are intended to help guide that thought process. I have also compiled chapter reflection questions at the end of each chapter to help you review your knowledge. Sometimes, reading these first can help prepare your brain for learning.

As you step into the role of working alongside a child as a therapist, teacher, or parent, you are now part of the collaborative group that will surround this child and collectively learn the best way to help them reach their potential.

At times, this book may feel overwhelming, but the goal is to open your mind to the possibility that there may be another side to what you see or hear. If you are a therapist, teacher, or specialist, recognize the value of engaging the parents or caregivers whenever possible.

If you are a parent reading this book and feeling overwhelmed, know that there are people out there who can help you and guide you through this process. You are not alone. Use the words and information in this book to help start the conversation of curiosity with others.

The stories in this book are based on some of the actual experiences I have had or heard while working with children, but the details have been changed to protect the privacy of those involved. I chose these stories because so many of the features of the stories will resonate with therapists, teachers, and parents alike because we all will recall children who had similar experiences. I use these stories to enhance your understanding of the knowledge I am speaking of in this book.

This is not a fully inclusive book of everything that makes up a child's story. Instead, it is a starting point to spark your curiosity and begin the conversation. I recognize there are limits to this book; there will be parts that may interest you, and you may wish to gain further information. At the back of the book, I have included a continued reading list for each chapter, highlighting some books that can dive deeper into the knowledge.

The ideas and suggestions contained in this book are not intended as a substitute for a professional working with a child.

Remember that you have an amazing opportunity to help a child unlock their potential and be seen for who they truly are. Together, we can watch these children take flight and soar!

Glossary/Abbreviations

Abstract Language	Using words that are vague with potential multiple interpretations
Affective Being	Emotional being or our feelings
CMOP-E	Canadian Model of Occupational Performance-Engagement
Cognitive Being	Ability to learning
Concrete Language	Words that have a specific meaning
Fixed Mindset	Have a set capacity for learning
Growth Mindset	Able to continue to learn and grow
Holistic Approach	Looking at all the pieces that can influence the outcome
IEP	Individualized education plan
Occupation	The activity or task a person wants or needs to do
PEO	Person, Environment, and Occupation Model
Physical Being	How we are physical made and interact with the world
Plan B	Actively involving the child in how to navigate a situation
Self-Regulation	The ability to manage stress and control emotions
Sensory Avoiding	Will often refrain from doing an activity with a certain sensory input
Sensory Craving	Will repeatedly seek out an activity that gives a certain sensory input
Sensory Overload	When too much sensory information is trying to be processed at one time
Sensory Preferences	A person's preferred input from the world around us
Sensory Room	A room that is often dedicated to sensory stimulating or calming activities
Tactile Defensive	Very sensitive to any touch

1   Introduction

Years ago, as part of an art class, the teacher showed me a black and white picture of a young woman. It was hand-drawn and was the outline of her face with a feather coming off her hair. The image was so clear to me, but half the class raised their hands when the teacher asked who could see an old woman in the picture. It was the cartoonist W. E. Hill's picture "My Wife and My Mother-In-Law" created in 1915.[1] As it turns out, in this drawing, the picture's perspective will change depending on your focal point. If you look at the smaller details, you can see a young woman, and if you look at the bigger details, you can see an older woman. Depending on how we are looking at the world, our experiences, perspectives, and focal points frame the way we see it. What fascinated me about this picture is that we were students in the same class, looking at the same drawing, seeing two different images.

How often do we experience this same story?

Have you ever watched a movie and walked out only to find out the person you went to the film with had a different experience in that same movie?

Or walked out of an exam thinking that was the most challenging test you had ever taken, only to hear your classmate tell you that it was so easy?

Have you ever felt misunderstood or wondered why people don't see life the way you do?

I am sure your answer is yes to one, if not all, of the aforementioned questions. Each person is looking at the world from their own perspective. This perspective is based on a number of factors, including where you were born, what era you were born in, who raised you, how you were raised, and all the experiences that you have had. Our perspective is formed from *our story*.

This book is about discovering your story and the story of the children we work with. It is about recognizing and understanding what influences our perspectives and the way we interact with the world. It is about putting down our technology and really engaging in the world around us. It is about helping children who are often misunderstood share their story. Too many times, we get caught up in the moment and what is happening in front of us, and we forget that we may not be seeing the full picture, just like in my art class.

DOI: 10.4324/9781003166405-1

Think about the experience of walking through a grocery store and seeing a child having a tantrum on the floor. People may judge the parent for not having control of their child.

Or the child in your neighborhood who runs around playing with no shoes on. People may think that this child is being neglected.

Think about a child who doesn't like to speak in public and shies away from groups. People may think that this child is depressed.

These are all examples of how our perception can influence the story we tell ourselves about these children and these situations.

Our own personal experiences, fears, emotions, and perspectives influence what we see. As you go through each chapter, you will be reminded of what other factors may influence a child's story and, in the same way, your story. We may not realize how differently our brains interpret the world through our sensory system, the way our minds process the information we learn, or the way we interpret a sense of belonging. The child in the grocery story may have been so overwhelmed by the sounds and the lights that he couldn't handle it any longer. The child running on the street without shoes may be oversensitive to socks and shoes, so he refuses to wear them. Each child's interpretation of the world is what makes them unique. It also makes each story important to share so that others can be more accepting of our differences. It is our unfolding stories that make this world a more interesting place.

Think for a moment what else can impact your perspective. If you were born before the Internet and before cell phones, when information was found at the library, or through talking with people. Imagine you were born in wartime, and you lived through the great depression, or a time when you had to practice bomb drills and hide under your desks. Or if, when you were little, you were not sure where your next meal would come from, or you worried for your safety when walking down the street. Think about the influence of social media and technology and how they have changed how we communicate and compare ourselves to others.

No matter how minor or extreme, each of these experiences could impact how you see the world today. They are part of what makes your story. It would affect what you value, appreciate, and what is important to you. It would also impact your worries, fears, and reactions.

These reactions can also affect how we raise or influence a child. I still recall when I was little that there were some friends whose parents would not let them make a mess within the home. Their home was always well kept and tidy. In that house, we had to constantly clean up behind ourselves as we went along, or we were afraid we would not be invited back. In other homes, you were not allowed to waste any food, so anything you had on your plate, you had to eat regardless if you were full or not. What were these parents' stories? What in their past formed their decisions with their children?

What was your childhood like? What influences formed your story?

When my children were little, they loved to get messy when they ate. I would often place some food pieces on their high chair's tray to encourage them to try and pick it up. I would even place some pieces of spaghetti on their tray. When they were learning, they would struggle to pinch the food, and it would oftentimes be smeared across their high chair. Sometimes, they would manage to pick up a piece and get it to their mouth, but by the end of the meal, they would be covered from head to toe with pasta sauce. Some would even end up on the floor. For some people, they may become upset with a child doing this and making a mess. Yet others may celebrate a child who has just learned how to feed themselves independently. Our response will be reflective of our own story, and how you react is based on your childhood experiences.

Sometimes, it is even just our instinctive reactions that can be a misinterpretation of a situation. I was in the process of potty training my child. We had been working on it for a while, and we were not having any success. Then one day, I hear from the upstairs hallway, "Mommy I went poo!" I ran upstairs and immediately saw a trail of droppings all the way down the hall, and there was my child standing naked in the hallway. Immediately, I got upset, as there was poo on the carpet. I started reminding them in a stern voice that we go on the toilet and not on the carpet and that they need to call mommy if they need to go. After my short rant, I carried them to the bathroom only to discover that they had gone on the toilet, and they were so excited that they immediately got off the toilet and ran to tell me. As a parent I felt horrible. My instinctive reaction was to be upset, when really I should have been celebrating their success. If we turn this story around and think of it from the perspective of the child, they are now confused, as they were being discouraged for something that they thought they were supposed to do.

We can be so quick to judge a situation when it all comes down to perspective. Understanding and looking at the whole story, not just what we see in front of us.

Discovering Someone Else's Story

Working with children involves the process of discovering and understanding someone's story. Discovering someone else's story can feel overwhelming, especially when it is not our child or a child we know. It can be even harder with a child who may not have strong communication skills. So where do you begin to understand a child's story?

Have you ever been in a bookstore and stood in front of a rack of hundreds of books, not sure which one to pick? We may pick up a book and look at the cover, and if the title or the picture interests us, we may flip it over and read the synopsis. If it doesn't interest us, we may put it back. Yet how much does the cover of a book actually tell us? As the saying goes, "never judge a book by its cover," which is true of books as much as it is true of people. How much can you really know about a person by just looking at them?

Just like when you start to read the story, you always begin at the beginning of the book. It is the same with understanding a child's story. You can't understand a child's story by how they look. You always start at the beginning of their story. Understanding who a child is involves understanding who is raising them and the environment that they are coming from.

Susie was a girl I worked with in Grade 1. She was referred for an occupational therapy consultation through the school system, as she was having difficulties staying focused at her desk, trouble with printing, and poor hygiene. Her teacher was concerned with how Susie looked when she came to school each day and was worried about how the other kids in the class were treating Susie.

When I met Susie for the first time, I was struck by the fact that in front of me was a 6-year-old girl wearing soiled clothes, with peanut butter in her hair, and smelling as if she hadn't showered recently. What I knew for a fact was that a 6-year-old does not come to school intentionally smelling poorly or wearing soiled clothes. She was not intentionally ignoring hygiene, which resulted in her classmates making fun of her and attempting to not sit close to her. There was more to Susie's story than what I could see from sitting with her at school.

Understanding first who was caring for Susie at home and their perspective was a key into Susie's story. When I connected with Susie's parents, I learned that Susie's mom was undergoing some medical treatments and had limited strength and mobility. To help out around the house, Susie was making her own breakfast and lunches to take to school. Susie didn't know how to do laundry on her own and had difficulty showering independently. They had some help in the house, but her mom didn't realize that Susie was wearing the same clothes to school each day.

Susie's story was an example of how a person's home life will affect school or community and vice versa. We can't separate a child from the impact of all the environments that they engage in. When we receive referrals from school, it often has school-related goals. School is a very different environment than home, but what happens at home can affect school.

Susie's struggle with focusing in class and printing her name had to do with what was going on with Susie at home. Understanding this part of the story helped me and the school staff work more effectively to support her at school.

Looking at Susie and the referral I received, many of the concerns focused on getting her to fit better into school. What those at school didn't realize is that Susie was trying to help out at home while her mom was undergoing medical treatments. Susie was doing more at home and for herself than many other 6-year-olds. With the family's permission, Susie was able to share with her class about what was going on with her mom. The perspective of Susie changed, and the class was able to learn empathy and think of ways to help Susie's family.

Many children have different experiences at home. Often, the first step is understanding the capacity of the family and how it can impact a child's story.

A child's ability to learn can be affected by the food that they eat, their genetic predisposition, and the nurturing that they receive. A referral for therapy should be about more than helping children to fit in better at school. Our goal is not only to make better students out of children; it is also about giving them the skills for a better future.

Can you relate to a story like Susie's? A child who is proud of herself for helping out at home, yet judged by others who didn't know the whole story. Susie smelt of peanut butter because she made her own sandwich for breakfast and had pushed her hair out of her face with her dirty hands. She had taken some creative initiative and showed independence to know what she needed to do before school, and that should be celebrated. How many of you reading this initially thought the case might be due to neglect? Sometimes, that can be our instinctive reaction, and we must always take a moment to think about what else could be going on. As you go through this book, I will outline in more detail all of the factors that can influence how we see and engage with a child. I will continuously emphasize the importance of always looking at the whole picture to help a child achieve their potential.

Understanding What Can Impact a Story

Once you understand where the story begins, it is also important to consider other factors that can be impacting how they behave. When children misbehave or have outbursts of emotion, there is often an underlying cause. Too often, I have watched children be disciplined for their behavior and see their behavior escalate out of control without taking the time to understand what caused the behavior. Our sensory system, our ability to learn, or an inability to regulate emotions can impact our reactions. I will go into detail in this book on how to recognize what could be impacting a child's behavior and what behaviors can tell us.

Luke was in Grade 3, was very disruptive in class, had difficulty focusing, and was labeled as a child with behavioral problems. Labelling a child can result in prescribing the fate of a child and I will go into this in more detail later in the book.

Luke was referred for occupational therapy to work on his classroom focus. During the first meeting with Luke, it was clear that Luke did have difficulty focusing, but that he also had trouble recognizing numbers and letters. When challenged, Luke would resort to acting silly or deviating from what was in front of him. At one point, he got up and tried to run away.

Luke didn't have many behavioral outbursts at home, but the environment at school had different expectations than at home. Luke was struggling with comprehension, recognizing letters, and fine-motor skills like printing, which was an obvious sign there was more to Luke's story than just the fact that he exhibited behavioral issues in class. He was struggling to understand and complete the work he had to do, which was a challenge.

If you or I were challenged with something as adults, at a task we not only didn't like to do, but also couldn't physically comprehend, would we stay willingly in that environment every day, or would we give up or try to get away? The negative perception that Luke was not behaving and acting out was missing many parts of that story. It was similar to Susie, who was judged for how she looked instead of looking at what else could be the cause.

Working through and identifying what made Luke who he is was such a valuable part of understanding how we could best support him. The sounds in the classroom and the discomfort of sitting in his chair were also making it hard for Luke to focus. His mind was focused on other aspects of the classroom, and therefore, there was a fight going on with the sensory inputs coming in around him. Each of the sensory inputs was trying to win the focus of the mind at that moment. Luke was feeling so overwhelmed that whenever anyone asked him a question or he had to try to work at his desk, he couldn't. When we were able to recognize the impact of the environment, we could make changes, including a few simple modifications in the classroom that would set him on the right track. We could then work collaboratively as a team around Luke to help him work towards his goal.

An important part of Luke's story is to understand that the feelings he was having were very real to him. The chair in the classroom may be fine for the other 23 students, but it was so uncomfortable for Luke that he couldn't concentrate. Luke didn't know how to express what he was feeling, so he would act out or just get up and leave.

I have often heard people use words like "This isn't hard" or "This can't bother you" when responding to a child's frustrations. Reframing this to acknowledging that these feelings and experiences are real for this child shifts our frame of mind, enabling creative solutions, positivity, and hope.

These two stories highlight some examples of why it is important to take the time to understand someone's story. Their stories give us a glimpse into what makes them who they are. This book is about identifying some of the pieces that make up a child's story. From before they were conceived, to the influences of the people who raised them, to the way that their brain interprets the world through their senses and how they learn, each part can impact how a child navigates the world. What we can recognize from their outward behaviors and the way they learn how to find balance is so important in a child's life. I hope that in this book you have personal ah-ha moments or takeaways that remind you that everyone has a story.

The most important part of this book is that each of us, no matter our role, title, or education, has the ability to uncover a child's story. Each of us is equally important and worthy of contributing to the success of a child. It is for this reason that I have written this book in a way that is applicable to therapists, educators, teachers, and health care professionals, as well as caregivers, parents, grandparents, camp counsellors, students, and anyone else who plays a role in a child's life. This book is written with the goal of helping anyone working with children or who has children to be able to look at the whole story of the child. In occupational therapy, we refer to this as a holistic approach—taking into consideration all their different components and parts. We owe it to the child to really grasp who they are and unlock their potential.

Understanding the Vision

Uncovering a child's story is so valuable, but it will only help if everyone recognizes the same capabilities of a child. If we were to try to help a child the way each of us thinks is best, we may not be as effective as if we work together and work towards a shared vision. So how do we work collaboratively together? What does this mean? How do we create a vision for a child?

A child's life can be thought of in relation to a sailboat. A sailboat is built for the water and with the intention to sail. If we tie a boat to a dock and let it stay there, it will not be used to its potential. Instead, we must learn about the boat, what makes it seaworthy, and how to let it reach its greatest capacity. The valuable information for a sailboat includes those who built the boat, the specification of the pieces that were put into it, and the environment it is in. What is also essential is how to sail the boat. The people who learn how to unleash the boat's capabilities will see the boat harness the wind and reach its potential. We cannot change what the boat is; we can only learn how to help the boat *do its thing*. The environment in which the boat will navigate will change, but when you understand the capabilities of the boat, you can move to environments that are favorable for the boat to fly through the water.

One would think that the sailboat's goal and vision are clear, but if the person who built the sailboat only wanted it to stay on dry land and the person who sails the sailboat needs it in the water, the vision is different. One is safe and secure, and the other is more vulnerable. Yet, in the water, you will see the most capabilities and learn the most.

Why compare children to boats? It is a clear example of a shared vision and goal. It shows the importance of understanding history as well as forecasting the future. It is about understanding the whole story and the bigger picture. It is about communicating these visions and goals with those around you effectively to become a shared entity. It is about learning to unleash the child's potential and focus on what they are capable of.

Having been a therapist working with kids and families in multiple settings, I have been involved with many different therapeutic relationship dynamics: meaning, I have worked with children, caregivers, teachers, other professionals, social services, and grandparents. What they all often have in common is their interest in the betterment of the child and their success. What I found different is that, sometimes, the goals and the approach varied. When there is no shared goal or vision for the child and no common understanding of the child as a whole, the outcomes can be altered. It is like we don't understand the boat and all its capabilities. This can come from a difference in our perspective. Understanding how to create a common vision for a child is important and covered later in this book. Once you have a vision, you can align all your goals towards the vision, which helps when making decisions about a child's future.

Sharing Someone's Story

As you uncover some parts of a child's story, it is important to think about how you would share your findings with others and be able to create a shared vision. How you share it can differ depending on the person you are sharing the information with, but the information is valuable so that a child is not misunderstood like Susie or Luke was.

Sharing a child's story reminds me of going to see a play. When you see a play at the theatre, you are given a program when you walk in. In the program, it tells you a little background or context to the play you are about to watch. It will tell you the setting, where the play takes place, and often the year that it takes place. It will also tell you the play's characters and a little background on who they are and the role they play in the story.

This information sets the stage for how the play will unfold and tries to create a common perspective for those watching. The screenwriter works hard to then create the scenes and the story to help us understand and relate to the characters. What makes each person who they are and how they contribute to the bigger picture is revealed as the play continues. We can see the emotion, the connection, the challenges, and the excitement as the play progresses. We are focusing on watching each move and the rest of story with anticipation.

In the unscripted play called life, we also have a setting and characters. Our setting is continuously changing, although many of the main characters will stay the same. There are specific roles and parts to the play that inform some of the background. The challenge with our life play is that we don't get the guide or program. We also don't get the benefit of rehearsals.

What if as therapists, teachers, parents, and caregivers, we use the information we discover about a child's story to create a guide or a program to help others to understand the children we work with? What if we create a way for people to understand a child's perspective, similar to a playwright describing characters in their play? Helping caregivers to find the language and express it to others empowers them and the children they work with to both be more active participants in their lives.

Working with children, no matter our role, title, or position, our goal is to support children through this ongoing play of life. Success comes from understanding what makes each character unique, leveraging their strengths, the setting in which life takes place, and how the characters interact with the environment that they are in. We are observing and learning more about the story of a child as it unfolds. Like a good playwright, as we learn more about each character and how they develop, we can work to create the settings that will help them to achieve their goals. The more we work at understanding ourselves and each other, the more we can enjoy and respond within our journey as care givers.

> *If you could write a description of your character in your play called life, what would it say?*
>
> *What would you be most proud of? What is your most significant ah-ha experience?*

As a mom, Susie's story, Luke's story, and so many more resonate with me and reflect the importance of understanding the larger picture and acknowledging the real struggle that children go through.

Don't we all wish we could be a little more understood by those around us?

Who these children are, not their diagnosis or label, but what they are capable of, is fundamental in helping them reach their goals. How kids learn or how they seek knowledge and information is so different from one child to another. We need to accept them for who they are and let them know that they are important and valued. By understanding the basics about how a child experiences the world through their senses, reacts through their behaviors, and learns through their unique style, we can create a future for them like no other. What if we could recognize what makes a child happiest? What if we could realize what makes them scared or sad? Then therapists and parents alike could create an environment that allows a child to thrive and flourish. Just like a flower in a garden, children are seeds: If planted in a supportive and enriching environment, this can help them thrive and grow.

To help you as a reader understand how the book was written, I will spend the next chapter explaining my perspective using an occupational therapy approach. Occupational therapy was built around a holistic approach to clients. Using models developed in occupational therapy can help guide us in processing the information we are dealing with. These theories provide us with a way to communicate a framework, helping take the whole story to identify the more specific parts and help in our approach to understanding children.

2 Occupational Therapy

To understand a child's story, you need to take a holistic approach. This means looking at all the pieces. As an occupational therapist, this is what we are trained to do. In this chapter, I am going to give you a glimpse of how occupational therapist thinking can help us go through the process of discovering what makes a child unique. Over many years of practice, occupational therapists, like many other professionals, have researched and developed guidelines, frameworks, models, and theories that help others within the profession to understand, navigate, and make sense of what we see. They help break down a big picture into smaller pieces, similar to how I described a child's story, and can help to give guidance on how to organize the information that we discover.

Why is this important?

Imagine sitting with 1,000 pieces of a puzzle in front of you, and you have no idea what image the puzzle makes. How do you know where to begin? Or if you were told to do a project at school or work without any guidance, direction, or expectations. Would you feel overwhelmed because you don't know where to start?

The key to conquering the feeling of overwhelm is by having a clear understanding or process of how to take a large task and break it down into smaller pieces. It is comparable to having the complete picture for your puzzle or an outline for the project that you need to get done. This guidance tells you how the pieces fit together or where you need to begin. That is what using an occupational therapy model can do. It can help us focus on all the parts that have been identified that affect who we are and what we do. This process drives results.

Think of this chapter as gaining the insight into my perspective and framing. I am sharing with you one of the perspectives that I use when I work with families and children. I don't just look at the small issues that might occur; I also look at the big picture: a holistic approach. There are different approaches, but for the purpose of this book, I want to keep it as clear and easy to understand so that we can share this perspective.

So, what is occupational therapy?

For those who know occupational therapy, you can skip ahead. For those who don't, here is a quick history lesson to describe what occupational therapists do and why occupational therapists think the way they do.

DOI: 10.4324/9781003166405-2

Numerous times, I have been told by a parent when I introduce myself as an occupational therapist that their child doesn't have a job yet. I always respond by saying that their job is to be a child, which we will work on.

Occupational therapy is often misunderstood because of its name. While people often assume the term occupational means it has to do with your job or occupation, the term occupation in the context of therapy has to do with any activity that a person participates in.

The therapy component works on exploring and answering many other questions around the activities. In relation to children, a few of which are:

Is the child able to do an activity that they want to do?
What is affecting their ability?
Can we help the child to reach their greatest potential in the activities that they want to do?
How can we make the activity more inclusive and accommodating to the child's needs?

A child's goal may be to learn how to ride a bike. They may be able to understand how to ride a bike, but the challenge is that they have difficulty balancing and controlling their legs. Since their goal is to ride a bike, I work with the child to find a bicycle that suits their needs. An accommodation might be that their bike may have three wheels, an increased back support, a wider seat, and some straps to hold their feet on. The occupation of the child at this moment is learning to ride the bike. The therapy is figuring out a way to help them reach that goal.

Occupational therapy came to be by understanding that there is more to a person than what we see in their actions. It is about finding ways to help people participate in meaningful activities. The models or guides help navigate each new situation to understand the people we work with and help them do the activities they want to do.

Where It All Began

We learn from history, as that is what informs the future. Here is a brief history of some ways that occupational therapy came to be.

The idea that we, as people, are designed and need to do purposeful, meaningful activities as part of our lives has been recorded back to the early 1800s. One example that is recorded is about a physiatrist named Dr. William Rush Dunton Jr., who worked in an asylum that housed people with mental health challenges that made them a danger to the community.[2] This came out of the era before we knew what we know now about how to help people. "Early in (Dunton's) work, he became intrigued by the healing potential of occupational activities for patients. His treatment recommendations included emphasis upon busy, productive activities in a patient's daily schedule."[2] Dunton published articles and books that emphasized the importance of meaningful work on healing the mind and body.

The occupational therapy profession continued to grow out of the need to find purpose and meaning for soldiers injured in the war.[3] Many soldiers wounded in the war were no longer able to serve in the military, and some could not return to the life they had before.

The soldiers went to war as healthy, capable humans who felt their purpose was to serve and protect their country. When they were injured, many struggled to find value and meaning in their lives. Yet these soldiers still had the capabilities to participate in meaningful work. Meaningful work was recognized as work that helps others and can contribute to the world's greater good.

Meaningful work is based on the idea that we are all created with the desire to have a purpose—a purpose in life to contribute, participate, and be a part of a bigger picture. When you cannot contribute in the way you originally intended or expected to, there can be a disconnect in life.

The early occupational therapists worked with soldiers to identify their capabilities and help them find activities in which they could participate. The occupational therapists looked at soldiers and recognized that they could still learn new skills, but their physical bodies were different. These early occupational therapists helped find ways to modify these soldiers' activities to allow them to be still independent. A simple example of an early occupational therapy goal was to create work that soldiers could sell. This work could even provide for their families—activities such as weaving baskets for soldiers who lost their legs in the war.[3]

The early practice looked at a person as a whole being, what they were capable of, what environment they were in, and how they interacted with their surroundings. How does someone learn how to navigate the world around them daily when physical or mental challenges exist? This idea grew into helping many diverse populations of people who face challenges in their daily lives. Modern-day occupational therapists continue to help solve the problems that interfere with a person's ability to do the tasks they want to do—everyday things like self-care, going to work or school, and any leisure activities.

Theoretical Foundation of Occupational Therapy

Over the last century, many frameworks, guidelines, theories, and models have been developed that create a way to help occupational therapists guide their strategies and ideas. Some are very specific to one area of practice, and others are broader.

So, what is the model or perspective used in this book?

The updated Canadian Model of Occupational Performance and Engagement (CMOP-E) created by Townsend and Polatajko[4] was designed to identify all the essential areas that effectively impact a person's ability to engage in a task. CMOP-E was one of many models based off a client-centered approach that many occupational therapists follow today. It helped to highlight how many factors affect a person's ability to complete a task.

There are three main areas of focus in the CMOP-E: environment, occupation, and person, and the core of this model is spirituality (Figure 2.1).

According to the CMOP-E model, a person, identified by the triangle shape, is a combination of affective, cognitive, and physical beings. Their physical ability: how they can move; their cognitive ability: how they can learn new ideas; and their affective being: how their emotions play into who they are, are all part of this model. The person triangle is built around the center core labeled as spirituality, not referring to religious affiliations, but that we, at our core, are unique beings.[4]

Through this model, the activities that we participate in are identified by the middle ring in Figure 2.1: (a) self-care, (b) leisure, and (c) productivity. Productive work for children would be any activity working to move a child forward on the learning continuum. Self-care activities are activities required of us daily, such as brushing our teeth, eating, toileting, exercising, and bathing. Leisure activities are those activities that we do for pleasure, such as sports, arts, and music.

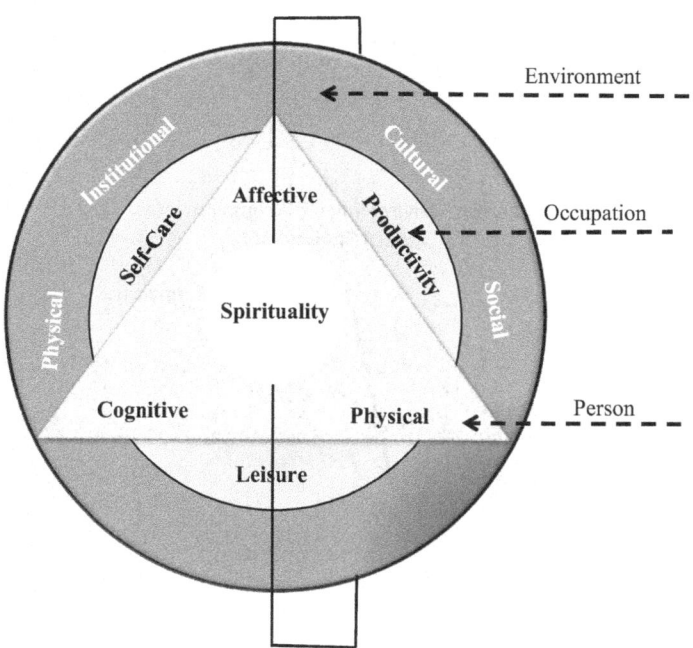

Figure 2.1 The three areas of focus in the CMOP-E in relation to its spirituality core.

Was directions for putting in the diagram

Note: Redrawn with permission from *Enabling Occupation II: Advancing an Occupational Therapy Vision for Health, Well-being and Justice Through Occupation* (p. 23), by E. Townsend & H. Polatajko, 2007, CAOT Publications ACE.

The outer ring of the CMOP-E model is the environment. The environment can be divided into four elements: the physical, institutional, cultural, and social elements (see Figure 2.1). The physical element would be any physical space that a child is in, including the tools and equipment that they use. The institutional elements include the law, rules, expectations, and practices that govern any environment. For example, how you behave in a church will differ from a school and differ from an art gallery, based on the rules or policies that govern this environment. The cultural element considers the cultural traditions that exist. This can include religious events such as Shabbat dinners in the Jewish faith on their sabbath Friday night. It can also include traditional activities such as sharing circles in the Indigenous communities, where the only person speaking has the talking stick, and you respect the messages and lessons that are shared. The social element of an environment includes all of the people who are within the environment that you are in. This can include family, coworkers, and friends whom you spend time with and can also include classmates, teachers, coaches, and even people who you may not know, such as at a store or park.[4]

It is important to take all three areas of focus and understand how they interact with each other. A simplified way to look at how the aspects of the CMOP-E model affect each other is through the Person, Environment, and Occupation Model by Law et al., also known as the PEO model.[5]

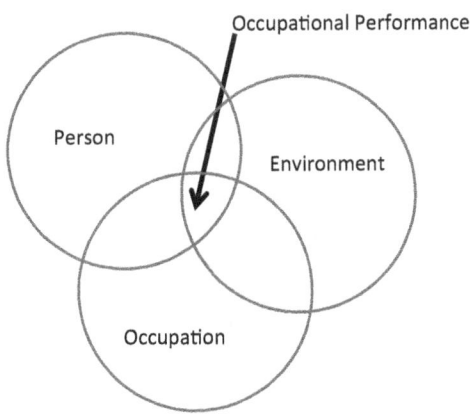

Figure 2.2 The person, environment, and occupational model.

Was directions for putting in the diagram

Note: Redrawn from "The Person-Environment-Occupation Model: A Transactive Approach to Occupational Performance," by M. Law, B. A. Cooper, S. Strong, D. Stewart, P. Rigby, & L. Letts, 1996, *Canadian Journal of Occupational Therapy, 63*, p. 18. doi:10.1177/000841749606300103

The basis of Law et al.'s PEO model[5] is that a person's performance can be evaluated in three areas: (a) the person, (b) the environment or where they are, and (c) what they do, also known as the occupation. When a **person** completes an **activity** in a specific **environment**, the result is known as **occupational performance**, or the result of the activity that was completed.

The more aligned the three circles are, the better the person will perform the task they are trying to do. Meaning that if the person has the skills to complete a task in an environment conducive to them doing the task, they are more likely to achieve it.[5]

For example, a child who has difficulty reading is easily distracted, and your job is to teach them to read. The child who has difficulty reading may have some sensory and attention challenges. The occupation or task they are trying to complete is the reading. The environment that you are working with them in is a rollercoaster ride. Because you are trying to teach them to read on a rollercoaster that has overwhelming sounds, movement, and sights, success in this task will be a challenge. The lack of success is because there is incongruence or disconnect between the environment and the activity you are trying to accomplish. The outcome of your job, to teach them to read, will likely not meet your anticipated goals.

If you were to take the same example of a child learning to read and were to move the environment to a quiet room, you would have better success working on their goal.

Sometimes, children may experience challenges working on skills in therapy sessions for this same reason. For example, when we teach children about dressing or toileting, but don't teach them in their environment where they would be completing the activity, such as a bathroom or their bedroom, they may have lower success in achieving the goal. According to Law et al.'s PEO model (see Figure 2.2), when the environment does not match the person and skill, that skill's outcome will be lower than expected.[5] It doesn't mean that the skills we can work on outside of this environment are not valuable. It is helpful to understand the model to know how to maximize the best outcome.

Similarly, suppose a child is not taught as part of their culture to feed themselves when they are young or to clean themselves in the bathroom. Even if we are in the proper environment, there would be a disconnect towards the goal. In that case, the cultural upbringing of the child affects the person in the model.

I worked with a little boy who was referred to me by the school system, as he wouldn't go to the school bathroom. It caused concerns for the school, as he would become irritable and anxious when he needed to have a bowel movement, and he often had to leave school to go to the bathroom. The school believed it was a fear issue, and they needed him to become more comfortable with toileting at school. When I spoke to his mom during the assessment, she described that she had never used toilet paper with her son. After he goes to the washroom, he takes a warm bath or has warm washcloths, and his mom wipes him down. She said that this was part of their cultural upbringing. Suppose a child understands that a warm bath is associated with going to have a bowel movement. In that case, the school environment will not allow him to complete the task the way he knows how to. There is no way to make the school environment more conducive to going to the washroom in this case. The challenge was not the boy's resistance to going to the bathroom. Instead, he was raised until this point to believe and understand that a warm bath occurs when you go to the bathroom.

Perspective

The school believed it was fear of the bathroom, and in some ways, it was. Yet there was more to this child's story that the school did not understand. When you look at the performance and not look at the pieces involved, you can be missing critical information that would affect the outcome.

The personal attributes did not match the environment, which affected the activity.

All three aspects (i.e., the environment, person, and activity) cannot be separated. Everything that makes up these components plays an essential role in creating our spirituality or what makes us unique. It may sound complex and a bit daunting, but if you understood the PEO model, think of these questions that can represent the details in the CMOP-E:

> *How do you act in different situations?*
> *Does the way you behave change depending on who you are with or where you are?*
> *Does the way you act change when you are not having a good day?*
> *Are some activities more comfortable to do than others? Or are there some activities that you would instead not do?*

The roles I play as a wife and mother are different from my role as a therapist. The location also varies greatly, with one being at home and one at a clinic. The way I communicate with my colleagues is different from the way I speak with my children. Understanding what factors are influencing me at any particular moment is essential, as it will impact what I am trying to accomplish.

It is all about perspective.

Understanding all the influences on a child is vital to work with each child effectively.

For example, consider the child I worked with who was unable to use the washroom at school. He could physically go to the bathroom. He was toilet trained. There was a disconnect in the environmental aspects between the cultural norms for his family, bathing after using the washroom, and the school's institutional requirements, using toilet paper. As therapists, understanding social and cultural influences on the environment is essential, as they can differ from person to person and from institutional norms or physical space. Understanding all of the child's story is necessary for creating a conducive space for growth and learning.

CMOP-E shows how many different factors affect a person's being and how unique each person is. Even two people raised in the same family will have two distinct sets of memories, emotions, and perspectives of the same activity. In the next chapter, I will identify some of the factors influencing those working with a child.

Other Professions

How is occupational therapy different from other professions? Models and frameworks are not just something that occupational therapists use. Many professions have created and practice under their own models and frameworks, which may impact the way they engage in the care of a child. We cannot assume that we understand each other's perspectives; therefore, it is important to be able to express our rationale and understanding of the situation. Acknowledging that differences exist, and how these may impact the outcomes of the interaction, is vital.

Think about the health practitioners you visit and the reason you go see them. You wouldn't go to a massage therapist for your child's pink eye. Likewise, you wouldn't go to a speech-language pathologist for help with walking.

More specifically, if you went to a family physician because you are struggling with anxiety, their focus and recommendations would be different than if you went to a social worker for the same reason. The amount of time spent, the depth of focus, and their treatment capabilities are different because of their professional training or focus.

When it comes to children, the training, expertise, and rationale that professionals are all taught serve the purposes they need in developing an understanding of a child. Each person plays a significant role in contributing information to the bigger picture. It is essential to understand the diversity in the perspectives and that everyone is looking at the same child from a slightly different angle. Think about W. E. Hill's picture "My Wife and My Mother-In-Law,"[1] which is the black and white image mentioned in the first chapter. The class members were all looking at the same image, yet we saw two different outlines.

Within each profession, there are also different specialties. A medical doctor can specialize in many areas: a cardiologist focuses on the heart, a radiologist focuses on medical imaging, a psychiatrist focuses on mental health, a pediatrician focuses on children, and the list goes on. Similarly, many therapists can work in different areas. An occupational therapist can focus their work on many areas, including seniors, children, hospital care, and home care. Although the overarching models used are the same, the treatment rationales, knowledge, and strategies can differ. An occupational therapist working with older patients in a nursing home would have a different experience than an occupational therapist working with children in a school setting. Both look at the clients similarly, but the client's influences, the environment, and the goals would differ.

Being aware of what professionals are involved in the care and support of a child and what perspective they have is important to understand how all the views and opinions fit together. Collaborating or working towards common goals can increase the chances of a successful performance of that activity. A speech-language pathologist working on bathroom vocabulary will impact a physical therapist helping a child work on balance in sitting, which will impact an occupational therapist working on the sensory needs as well as the sequence of toileting. Although each person's focus was on a different part, together they worked on the larger goal of independent toileting.

Occupational Therapy in Pediatrics

When people see an occupational therapist working with children, they often see pictures of children on swings or playing on the floor. Sometimes, images will show children building with blocks or working on letters. Yet an occupational therapist does so much more.

A child's job is to learn and grow from experiencing the world. We work with children and their parents and caregivers to learn and identify how each child experiences and navigates the world. Occupational therapists are like detectives gathering all the information surrounding a child, as outlined in the CMOP-E,[4] to understand the challenges children face. We then work to help children develop skills or ways to work towards specific milestones created from observing children's natural progressions. This looks different for each child, but the more we understand about a child's needs and preferences, the better we can support a child to flourish. An occupational therapist's goal is to help children maximize their independence in their occupation of play, develop their self-care skills, and achieve their greatest potential in home, school, and community.

Occupational therapy was born out of helping people find purpose and meaning. Using models like the ones reviewed in this chapter gives us a framework of how to identify what part or area may be having an impact on the other areas. We can use these models to also identify the influence of anyone working with a child. Each of us, even as parents, caregivers, and professionals, can learn about our natural biases, experiences, and mindset and how these can impact our decisions. This is the starting point for the next chapter because when we first understand more about who is raising the child, we can understand more about how a child might view the world.

Chapter Reflections

1. What is the value in following a model when working with children?
2. What are the two models we looked at in this chapter that will guide the rest of this book?
3. How do the person, environment, and occupation relate?
4. Why is it important that all three factors align?
5. Why is it important to understand other professions, models, or frameworks?

3 Understanding the Caregiver

Have you ever thought about when a person's story actually begins? When you tell someone about yourself, do you talk about your life as it is now? Do you start when you were born? Or do you start from where your parents were born?

The person or people who are raising a child and the environment that a child is raised in create the setting for the first part of a child's life. Yet, when we think about a child's story, we often don't start the discussion by looking at who the caregivers are.

The truth is that every child's story begins before they are born. There is a large biological component to who we are. What happens after we are born—where, how, and who raised us—then impacts how our traits develop. This is important because how we were raised forms our values, beliefs, and views of the world and ourselves. What a person learns when they are growing up will impact how they interact with the next generation. Seeking to understand how a child is raised can help us to know how to unlock their potential.

The information about a caregiver can help give clues into the parts of a child that they can't communicate yet. As you go through this chapter, think about your own experiences and how it may impact the way you see the world today.

Grade 7 Biology

What makes a person who they are includes one's physical, cognitive, and affective being as highlighted by Townsend and Polatajko in their CMOP-E.[4] Many of these features can have genetic links.

If you think back to Grade 7 science class, a person (a new life) is created when two cells combine half the DNA from one person and half the DNA from another. Through this process, an entirely new human being is created. The people who created this tiny human have given the starting blocks for how this child looks, grows, and develops. Research has shown many different traits can be determined through the genetic makeup we are given from

DOI: 10.4324/9781003166405-3

our biological parents. Biology sets some of the groundwork for who we will become.

Why are genetics important?

The key to understanding parts of the child can come from understanding their biological parents.

What kind of struggles did the parents have as children?
What were their strengths? Sensitivities? Challenges?

In more recent years, scientists have discovered genetic links to traits such as focus, attention, and sound sensitivity. Knowing some of the genetic makeup only gives us clues into how a child functions. We need to remember that children are not identical replicas and, therefore, will not be the exact same as their parents. When I thought about having children, I always believed that I would have mini versions of myself. We would be interested in the same activities and have similar personalities. I would know exactly how they wanted to be parented on the basis of my own experiences. It would be easy. This was far from the truth. As a mom of four beautiful children, I can say that they are all unique and individual, and **not one** is like me. I learned so much from each, including how to see them as unique individuals and to parent them all differently. It was not the easy experience I was hoping for. They did, however, carry on some of those traits that are biological. The importance of these factors in a child's development can give us some clues into what makes the child who they are.

Understanding How You Were Raised

Part of who we are is made up of this genetic component, and the other piece is how we were raised. When we look at who is raising the child, we can see a different set of characteristics that may affect a child. The person caring for a child can vary from the biological parents, grandparents, extended family members, foster parents, adopted parents, and guardians. At any point in time, there is a person legally responsible for caring for that child.

Since there are no mandatory courses on how to raise a child or care for a child, the information that we have on how to raise children comes mostly from our own experiences. This includes information from how we were raised, how we saw others around us raised, stories we were told, and what we saw on television and social media. Think about the families that lived near you growing up. Did you sometimes think about what it would be like to be part of another family? Did you see a show on television and wish your parents could be like those characters?

Each caregiver's story is influenced by the environment (i.e., physical, institutional, cultural, and social) they were raised in, as noted by Townsend and Polatajko in their CMOP-E.[4]

The physical elements of the environment that you grew up in shaped your experiences. Think about the last 100 years and how much the physical world has changed. From the beginning of the 20th century to the end, the world looked like a much different place. With the evolution of transportation, the world became a much smaller place. People could travel more easily, and families became spread out across the globe. What used to take weeks to travel, now with air transportation, only takes hours. From the introduction of the television to the technology we have access to today is drastically different. With the growth of the World Wide Web, access to unlimited information is now at our fingertips. Even the influences of the media have changed how children in the 21st century will grow up. We can see and compare ourselves to so many more people than ever before. People far removed from our lives can even comment on the way we live our lives based on images that they see on social media.

On a smaller scale, the physical community you grew up in, the schools you attended, and the homes you have lived in will have created memories and experiences that have become part of you. Even the bedroom you had, the toys you played with, and activities you participated in informed your being. Your feeling of safety, your sense of support, and your understanding of community were formed in these younger years. Someone brought up in a refugee camp with very little will have a different outlook than someone who grew up with everything they ever wanted or needed. A family who lived in poverty, not knowing where the next meal would come from, would understand hardship more than someone who didn't. A family who lived through the war where they were afraid to leave their house may be more aware of the freedoms of where they are now living than someone who has not experienced war. All of these physical elements will impact who we become.

The social elements are also important to understand as it would include all of the people that were part of your childhood story. Who was around us when we were growing up would have impacted what community meant to us.

Think about Sarah: a little girl who was an only child raised in a home where her mom stayed at home and cooked, cleaned, and made sure she was taken care of. Sarah's dad worked out of the house and would be gone from nine to five, come home for dinner, and spend his evenings reading the paper or watching television. There were strict rules in the house for Sarah: no television, music, yelling, or talking back. There were very few words of affirmation or hugs. Sarah was considered a good child if she obeyed the rules and did well at school. She was only allowed to play with a few neighbor children, but was not close to any relatives. She was given anything she wanted as long as she stayed quiet. Sarah will grow up with the social and emotional influence of this upbringing. Her sense of acceptance and love will affect how she will approach motherhood and how her children will be raised. Even if she disagreed with how she was brought up, many of those emotional ties and social influences would affect her future experiences.

Another example would be a little boy named Sean, who had two siblings, raised by a single mother. His mother couldn't work because of a disability, and so they lived on social support. It meant that his family relied on government aid as a resource for income for food and living. His mother gave him lots of hugs, encouragement, and love. He had few resources at home, but he knew he was loved. Sean never had the newest clothes or the latest toys, but his mom always told him he could be whoever he wanted to be. He had cousins, aunts, and uncles involved in his life, and he was part of a large extended family unit that he often saw. His family was also part of a nurturing faith community. These experiences will influence his role as a parent.

These two children will grow up with different social experiences, which will influence how they parent. These examples are only two of millions of other stories. No two people are going to have the same experiences. Even children from within the same family will have different emotional responses and memories to the same event.

The cultural elements in our childhood include those traditions and values based on the generations before us. Each family has a family culture, which can be a mix of cultures brought together through marriage or relationships. The way your family celebrates holidays, its religious associations, and traditions will influence what you value as an adult. It doesn't mean you will carry on these traditions necessarily, but the way you interpret your experiences as positive or negative will determine how they affect your adult life, and this outcome will ripple into your children. If Thanksgiving was an important family holiday each year with a big dinner and lots of family, you may want to continue this tradition if it brought you joy when you were a child.

The institutional elements of your upbringing can be reflective of many different areas. It can include the country that you grew up in and the rules, laws, and societal standards that existed within it. I believe that institutional influences go beyond the government and include any environment where rules or regulations exist. This can include any rules that occurred in your home from your parents. This can also happen in any association, religion, educational, or professional environment. Think about a team's organization. There are rules embedded in participation in their programs, and there are expectations of behaviors. The school you went to as a child would have had its own rules, position on behavior tolerance, and discipline. What happened when rules were broken and how the school dealt with it may have impacted your future educational experiences and opportunities. Even working as an occupational therapist, there are rules that govern how I can work, communicate about my profession, and behave that will affect my choices throughout my career. These rules create boundaries and potential limitations that will impact the choices you make. These institutional elements will affect how you have grown up.

Take a moment to think about your childhood:

>   *What was your family home like?*
>   *What were some experiences that you enjoyed?*
>   *Who were the important people in your life?*

How you answer those questions will often impact how you approach the children you work with or your own children. Our experiences growing up are what we relate our current situation to. If we had a difficult childhood, we may think that children today have it easier. What we need to recognize is that each era and generation has its own challenges, and only you know what you have experienced in the past. Our experiences create perspectives on how we view the world and our expectations within the world.

Impact of Life Experience

Sometimes growing up, we wish we were given different opportunities. We can wonder how our life would have been different. This can affect the choices we make as adults and parents.

Sam had always wished he had played competitive hockey. He thought that if he had been able to get more training and compete at higher levels, he would have been able to go further with a hockey career. His parents didn't encourage him and couldn't afford it. As a parent, Sam doesn't want to get in the way of his son competing in hockey and gives him every opportunity to play at higher levels and have extra training. Sam may be more likely to push his child harder because of his own dreams and desires.

This could also happen when you want a child to keep up with others. Such as a parent who wants their child to be as successful in math as the child down the street and puts them in hours of tutoring to help them keep up, even if math is not their child's strongest skill.

We need to understand what our goals are versus what is best for our child. What part of your own story is impacting how you see a child? In her book *The Conscious Parent*, Dr. Shefali Tsabury stated that when we are aware of our parenting, "We have to become astute observers in our own behaviors when we are with our children. In this way, we can begin to be aware of our unconscious scripts and emotional imprints."[6]

It is not just how you were raised. It can even be something that happened to you when you were a child that impacts your reactions as an adult.

I was bullied in grade school. I have three older brothers who taught me how to play sports, and I loved every minute of it. When it came to recess at school, I would choose sports with mostly boys over walking around with the other girls in the class. Even though this is who I was, I became ostracized or excluded by the other girls. They called me names, would laugh behind my back, and wouldn't talk to me. I would often come home crying from school. A child wants to feel included and a part of something, and the girls in my class made it hard to feel that way.

Being bullied made me extra sensitive as a parent to what my children might be facing at school. I remember what that felt like—not wanting to go to school the next day, scared to go out for recess, feeling alone. I never wanted my kids to feel that way. I didn't want any other children to face this either.

My experiences as a child influenced how I react to situations as an adult. When I hear about children experiencing what I experienced, I have an immediate reaction that triggers my past emotions. I recognized this when my oldest came home from school and told me he was picked on by another kid in his class every recess. My initial reaction was anger and an attempt to protect my son from experiencing what I experienced. I am conscious that my past was influencing my ability to see the situation in front of me. When I spoke to the teacher, I needed first to acknowledge that I was bullied as a child and am sensitive to children being picked on. When I explained my perspective, it allowed the teacher to understand the emotional response I had to this situation. I recognize that my reactions may be different from someone who has never experienced this before.

It doesn't even have to be about something that happened to you. The experience can be something you attended or witnessed that became stored in your memories and has affected your future choices. Think about

> *The first wedding you went to.*
> *The first baby you held as a child.*
> *The first funeral you attended.*

What you were exposed to as a child will shape your understanding of life in general. I attended my first funeral when I was in Grade 1. Until this point, I had never really discussed death or thought about death. I remember many moments from that day, and those memories impacted choices I have made since that moment.

Our exposure to life experiences growing up will also influence our comfort in working with people with differing needs. An occupational therapist who grew up in a home with a sibling who had physical differences will understand what it means to make accommodations for them in the home more than someone who didn't have such experiences. They may have had to help take care of their sibling and understand the challenges they encountered. This therapist may be able to relate to a child they are working with who has similar challenges.

A social worker whose parent struggled with depression, who couldn't get out of bed to make meals, or was unable to help with homework or be involved with her activities will have a different understanding of the effects of depression on children.

Our life experiences become part of our story and shape our understanding and empathy of situations, which can ripple down to affect the children we work with.

A teacher who did well in school, was liked by all their teachers, needed very little help, and loved doing homework may have different expectations for their students than a teacher who struggled through school, especially if the second teacher was considered to have a behavioral problem, was always in trouble, and had little family support. Additionally, consider a teacher who had children of their own who feared school and had to work tirelessly to help their child succeed. What each person experienced growing up will impact how they view and treat others and will affect their perspective in working with their students.

Carter struggled with anxiety at school. He feared any form of testing and felt that if he got any questions wrong, that people would think he was incompetent. Therefore, he had anxiety leading up to tests, the thought of tests, and then sitting with the test in front of him. Carter knew the information on the test, but the idea of getting the answers wrong made him so afraid that he sometimes could not even answer the questions. His mind would go blank. He was too afraid to raise his hand to ask for the teacher's help, as he didn't want others to know he was struggling. Instead, he would sit till the end of class and hand in a nearly blank test. Anxiety can be hard to understand. For Carter's Grade 5 teacher, her son had struggled in the same way. She knew the fear that her son had and how it impacted his experience. So, this teacher would allow Carter to come in during recess when the room was quiet and give him more time. She did not penalize him for his blank test; instead, she would encourage him and reassure him to show his abilities, even if the answer was incorrect. His teacher's personal experience had impacted her empathy for her students.

The experiences of therapists and teachers affect their perspectives and potential expectations of the children in their class or the children they work with. It in turn affects how children are received and how they are seen. Carter knew the information, but was so stressed he couldn't get the information out. Another teacher may have assumed that Carter didn't study for the test. Two very different perspectives on the same situation.

The negative experiences people have can also create trauma points in life that can trigger emotional and physical responses that will alter how they experience the world from that point on. What people said to you or how they described you or your life could have long-term effects, reflected in words like failure, no good, useless, intolerable, incompetent, ugly, or unlovable. Negative words that we believe can make us think that we are incapable of success in our lives. Suppose that there is any history of physical, emotional, or sexual abuse from an adult in a child's life. In that case, this can impact any future relationships and how the child relates and trusts other adults in their life.

Why is this important when looking at a child's needs?

The experiences we have as a child and how we were raised have such a profound impact that we can't ignore them. We need to recognize that these impacts are not just what happened to us, but they can also result from something that happened to the people who raised us. The cycle can go back from generation to generation. We all have a story.

When working with children, it is essential to be aware of the caregiver's impact and all those events surrounding that child's experiences and perspectives. How do you assess this? Use your observation skills, and watch as the parent interacts with the child. Ask questions about the caregiver's upbringing, especially as it relates to the child's needs. Have they experienced something similar to what their child is going through? How would their caregiver have dealt with this situation when they were little? Sometimes, we are not aware of what is impacting our choices, but there are often clues that can help us unlock them.

Capacity

Beyond the story of a caregiver's childhood and how they were brought up is their current capacity, which can also influence a child's day-to-day experiences, and the capacity of a caregiver can change from day to day.

> *Have you ever been upset about something going on in your life and then tried to console others at the same time?*
> *Have you noticed what happens to the mood in the room when someone is angry?*

The atmosphere changes.

As a parent, if I am upset about something that has happened, I have less patience, am more irritable, and my children can sense that. It also changes the way that they react to any situation. I recently had a bulging disc in my back. I couldn't sit, stand, or even laugh without pain. For a child who sees you in pain, there are many ways that they can react. My one son became timid and wary of coming near, more for fear of making my pain worse. My daughter became clingy, worried for me, and did not want to leave my side. My other daughter became extremely helpful with making food, tidying up, and caring for me. My children were scared, and it affected how they treated each other. A small child does not understand your pain, your struggles. They can only sense how this reflects on them. A child may not be able to console an adult or even show empathy yet, as they may not be at that stage of development. What the child can sense is the change in the connection.

If a parent or caregiver struggles with emotional or mental health issues or even physical pain, their capacity to be present for a child is altered during that time. Loss of a job, a new diagnosis of cancer, death of a loved one, or any of these examples of life changes can affect our energy and ability to be present for our children. A child can sense changes in this connection, and a child may begin to seek attention and connection in other ways. Think about Susie in our first chapter; her mom was undergoing medical treatments that made it hard for her to help Susie. Sharing this knowledge with the class changed their perspective and how Susie was treated in the school. Many times, being open about what a caregiver is going through can allow others to have greater empathy and support for the child.

Connection to the Child

The connection created and experienced between the caregiver and the child is the bond that can impact the emotional, cognitive, and mental development of the child. How a caregiver interacts with the child can have lasting impacts on how the child interacts with the world. What a caregiver says or how they treat the child influences what a child believes about themselves. The caregiver's perspective on a child can be influenced, as discussed previously, by the way that caregiver was raised, the era, and the experiences they had.

The connection can also be affected by the child's abilities. The more a child differs from the caregiver, the more challenging it can be. If a child struggles physically, mentally, or emotionally, it can be hard to find that connection, especially when the expectations for a child differ from how they are born and develop. Think of Sam, who wanted his son to be a hockey player. If his son was born with physical limitations so he couldn't play hockey, the disappointment that Sam may have felt could have affected the connection he had with his child. Creating a bond with a child for who they are is an integral part of a child's sense of acceptance, love, and comfort and will help them reach their potential.

> *Think about a person in your life growing up that you felt connected to.*
> *What characteristics did they have?*

A genuine connection develops with someone who takes the time to understand a child, sees the child for who they are, not the product of their behaviors—just like Carter's homeroom teacher, who understood that Carter's anxiety was not defining who he was. It was only a part of who he was, and she had the opportunity to help him learn how to manage it. The homeroom teacher's connection to Carter can drastically impact his anxiety. If Carter was afraid of the teacher and her reaction, this can increase his school anxiety. If a teacher supports them through it, understands a child's needs, and loves them no matter what, a child can sense this and would be more likely to gain confidence in himself and decrease anxiety.

When the connection is not present, it can have negative impacts. Carter's music teacher was not the same as the homeroom teacher. She would only come in twice a week to the class to teach music. She didn't have as much time to get to know the students, so she never really connected with them. Carter did not like to play in front of the class, nor did he like to be called out in class from the teacher. On one particular day, Carter forgot to bring his instrument to school. He never forgot his instrument because he knew what happened if you did. The teacher would call you out in front of the class and make you use one of the extra instruments she brought in with her.

Just as he thought, the music teacher asked everyone to take out their instrument at the beginning of the class. When Carter realized he did not have his instrument, the teacher requested Carter to come to the front of the class and get one of the extra ones she had brought along. What happened at that moment was that Carter's anxiety and fear took over, and he couldn't move. He was angry at himself for forgetting his instrument, and he was embarrassed about having to get up in front of the class. The teacher didn't know that Carter's anxiety was so high that it affected his ability to think about anything other than finding somewhere safe to go. She demanded he come to the front of the class, but instead, all Carter could do was put his head down on his desk. After multiple attempts, the teacher continued with the class.

The music teacher had called Carter's mother after the class to inform her of Carter's disrespect for the teacher and his unacceptable behavior. What was more shocking to the teacher was the mother's response, which informed her of the high anxiety experienced by Carter. The teacher was also told how long it had taken Carter to build enough self-regulation to know that he had to put his head down to remain calm and composed. If he didn't do this, he would have run out of the classroom crying and further escalated the situation into something more significant, which was the basis for previous bullying by other students. This teacher never called out a child again to the front of the class, and Carter never forgot his instrument. Her perception had been that he was disrespecting her. This may have triggered something in her that made her fearful of losing control of the classroom or of not being respected. This may be part of the music teacher's story, and anxiety was part of Carter's story.

The difference between the homeroom teacher and the music teacher is that one connected with Carter and took the time to understand and create a safe and supportive environment. The other did not build that connection and may have rushed to conclusions, unaware of the entire picture. One helped Carter to decrease his anxiety, which, in turn, allowed him to build the strategies that will impact him in the future. The other increased his fear and anxiety.

How do you create a connection?

There are many ways to create a connection between a child and a caregiver. The most effective way is to be present with the child (i.e., physically, mentally, and emotionally present). This means that as a caregiver, you listen to them as they share their stories, without interrupting or quickly judging. You physically sit close to them and look them in the eyes. Get to know the child's abilities, challenges, and fears. Show interest and enthusiasm or concern for their stories, activities, movements, acceptance of where the child is, and how they perceive the situation.

Mindset

Throughout this chapter, we have learned what impacts a person's story and how it can affect how we see the children in our lives. These include the biological and environmental influences as well our life experiences and current capacity. What we believe about ourselves and what we believe about others will impact our relationships in the future.

There are two different ways to think about ourselves and our abilities as we move through this book. In her book *Mindset: The New Psychology of Success*, Carol Dweck highlighted that if you believe you were born with "only a certain amount of intelligence, a certain personality, and a certain moral character,"[7] then you have a fixed mindset. In essence, it would be like saying you're not a good golfer after your first time playing, and you never return to play. As a caregiver, an example of a fixed mindset would be that you believe that your child by age 10 is as smart as they will be. However, if we take this information that we learned about ourselves and those around us and believe that what we have experienced and learned is just the starting point for development, it is called a growth mindset.

> The growth mindset is based on the belief that your basic qualities are things you can cultivate through your efforts, your strategies, and help from others. Although people may differ in every which way—in their initial talents and aptitudes, interests, or temperaments—everyone can change and grow through application and experience.[7]

With a growth mindset, if in your first golfing game you did poorly, but believed that you could do better, you would practice, hire a coach, keep playing, and improve.

Our mindset can impact our belief in ourselves and our capabilities working with children. If you believe you know all you need to know, then you have a fixed mindset. If you believe that there is a world of information that can help you improve and grow in your knowledge, then you have a growth mindset. This book is about gaining a new understanding of the children we work with, and my hope is that this book will help you see a different perspective which will inspire you to a new level of curiosity.

Caregivers can also think of their children through these two types of mindsets. If they think of a child through a fixed mindset, they would believe that a child has limited potential and that they can't go beyond that potential. This can often happen when a diagnosis is given, and they are told the limitations of the diagnosis. A child who can't speak and a caregiver who is told they will never communicate may look no further into opportunities. A child who can't walk may be told their future opportunities are limited. Yet both of these are examples of a very narrow fixed mindset.

Michael struggled in school and had been diagnosed with a learning disability. His high school teacher took him aside and told him that he would not do well in the business world if he didn't do well in her class. Her inability to see the growth beyond her class could have been discouraging for him had it not been for others who saw him differently.

With a growth mindset, the child would be viewed as having endless potential. The caregiver believes that the child is not limited by their diagnosis, but is considered a person with unlimited opportunity. Michael had other teachers who took the time to understand him, asking questions that enabled him to continue pursuing his learning and work on his strengths. Michael came to know that if he continued to work hard, he could achieve more. A child who can't speak, if given the right opportunities, may create brilliant speeches. We don't want to be the limiting factor in a child's life.

When working with caregivers, it is crucial to understand their belief in themselves and their child's abilities, identifying their mindset.

> *What is your mindset?*
> *Do you believe that people can continuously grow and develop?*
> *Do you believe in your capabilities to help the child, and are you willing to learn if you don't know something?*

We all have a story. What makes up our story and those of the caregivers of the children we work with, including the environment and experiences, will influence how we interact with a child. Our story can impact a child's story. Yet our story will always be different from a child's story, and we need to make sure that we try our best to be open minded when focusing on the child. Having a mindset that believes in a child's potential will keep your eyes open to opportunities to support a child and help them reach their goals. As we proceed through the rest of the book, we will take an in-depth look at how to understand a child's story from the child's perspective. When we gain this insight, we can learn how to advocate for and support a child in a way that best meets their needs.

Chapter Reflections

1. Why is it important to understand who is raising a child?
2. How can genetics impact a child's development?
3. What is the difference between physical and social elements of the environment?
4. Why is it important to understand your background when working with a child?
5. What is the difference between a fixed and growth mindset?

4 Understanding the Child

Sometimes as adults, we may think we know what a child's story is before we have even met them. Parents may make assumptions about one of their children based on their personal experience or in comparison to their other children. This happens without even realizing it.

I had a job as a swimming instructor when I was in high school. I loved teaching children how to swim. I loved the water, and when children came for swimming lessons, I felt my job was to help them see how fun the water could be. Since it was a community pool, we would get the same children returning every session for lessons. Children would move from instructor to instructor as they moved levels or stayed at the same level. The odd time, you would get a child who was just terrified of the water. The past instructors would warn you about them, and before you even saw the child, you would be prepared for the fight.

That was the problem. The child didn't get the chance to meet me without me already making judgments or assumptions about who this child was and how this session would go.

Preconceived judgments happen in so many aspects of our society. Think about a therapist receiving a chart with a child's diagnosis or concern on it, or a teacher learning from another teacher what to expect from a child entering their class in the new year. What about a sports coach warning about a child who will join their team or the fear of having a sibling of a child in your group who had previously caused chaos in the same group?

We can make assumptions about a child before we even get a chance to see them.

My daughter was very active in school and had difficulty focusing on the task at hand. She would get distracted easily and often wanted to see what others were doing. Repeatedly, she would be told to sit at her desk. She would return only to be up moving around again shortly after. Other girls in the class didn't like it when she was coming up to them. My daughter was labeled the "mean girl" in class by one of her teachers. This label followed her for a couple of years. Each year, the teacher would send notes home discussing her inability to focus and her being unkind to other kids in her class.

DOI: 10.4324/9781003166405-4

It wasn't until she reached a teacher that didn't focus on what other teachers had said about my daughter. Instead, she focused on what she saw in class for herself. She looked at her strengths and abilities, kindness towards others, creativity, and helpful nature. This teacher encouraged kindness. At the parent–teacher interview with this teacher, she had only positive reviews and even mentioned that she didn't see any of the traits she was warned about. That teacher's ability to focus on our daughter's strengths drastically changed our daughter's school experience that year.

It was almost as if our daughter had a clean slate that year. Someone took a moment to look at who she was, not the result of what she had been previously.

Have you ever wished to be seen for who you are now, not what you were in the past?

It is crucial to spend time with a child to explore the facts, not what someone has told us. As we discussed in the previous chapter, some of the facts include that a child is a biological product of two people with the nurturing influence of their caregivers. As we continue to move through this book, I will highlight the characteristics that make each child unique. Since a child's story is continually changing, it is important for them to be seen for who they are at a given moment rather than what they were in the past.

Johnny was a little boy who had difficulty focusing in the classroom. He was often disruptive, moving around, and would often get into other people's space. He was identified as a behavioral concern in the school and was often sent to the office. His teacher started the year prepared for the challenge his presence would entail, just from the stories she had heard. His teacher viewed Johnny as disruptive and undisciplined. Johnny also loved to do gymnastics and had just become a member of the local gymnastics club. At the gymnastics club, he was energetic, disciplined, and eager. The coaches loved working with him, as he was always willing to try something new.

Do you see the difference in perspective from one caregiver to another?

Johnny is the same child; so why does Johnny respond differently to different environments?

Some of it may come from the interactions with the caregiver in each situation. His teacher expected that Johnny would be disruptive and exhibit "behaviors." Therefore, whenever he did, she was right on it. His gymnastics coaches didn't have the expectation that Johnny was a behavioral problem or disruptive. When they met him this season, they only saw how he engaged in the class, how talented he was on the floor, and how he worked with others. The caregivers' past experiences, biases, and expectations, or lack thereof, set Johnny up for how he was treated in each environment. Such preconceptions can affect the relationship between the child and the caregiver.

Instead, when working with a child, we need to fully understand what makes a child who they are. Looking at a child from the perspective of their physical components, their affective beings, and their cognitive beings, as described in the model we reviewed called the CMOP-E covered in Chapter 2, can give us clues into what makes a child unique.[4]

Physical Being

A child's physical abilities cover a wide range of subcategories about how a physical body interacts with the world around it. The way our bones and muscles are formed to the way our nerves connect to these structures and how our brain processes information can all differ from person to person.

We should never make assumptions about a person based on their physical appearance or the way a physical body works, as appearance and differences do not define one's abilities. Amazing art has been created by people who are blind or who have no hands. Incredible stories have been told by people who cannot speak.

Remember, it is not about a child being like us, or the same as another child or how the world thinks a person should be. *It is about what a child can bring to the world.*

To understand a child's physical abilities, they need to have the opportunities to explore the world. How does a child interact with the world? I once heard a motivational speaker by the name of Nick Vujicic talk about his life. He was born without arms and legs, but despite the challenges he faced, he could find ways to navigate the world in his own way. He described learning to stand by using his chin as a brace against the wall. If he was not given a chance to try this, he might have never learned how to transition from lying down to standing independently.[8]

Our physical bodies also include how we process information through our physical structures. How do children use their senses to experience the world? How does a brain interpret sensory experiences? The body is made up of eight unique sensory systems that interact with each other and send signals to the brain to inform and interpret the world around us. Each person can have such unique experiences with the sensory information, and this can affect how they function in the world. It is such an important part of what makes us unique that I will spend the next chapter going into more details.

Affective Being

Beyond our physical being is our emotional being or our feelings. One of the most essential points is: What makes a child feel like they belong and are connected? What makes them feel loved? How do they experience the world?

In her book, *Positive Discipline*, Jane Nelsen spoke about needing to feel that you belong to a larger purpose and play some significance in that purpose, which are goals for all people, especially children.[9]

A child not chosen to be a part of a soccer team at recess or a child made fun of because of their clothes may not feel like they are part of the group. A teacher who never calls on a child in class or a parent who ignores their child and constantly scrolls on their phone may make a child feel lonely or unwanted. A doctor speaking poorly about a child when a child is present may make that child not feel accepted. These scenarios all create the sense for a child that they don't belong or are not valued.

Was there a time when you didn't feel like you were part of a group?

When I was little, I was the youngest of five children. The four oldest were very close in age, and there was a gap between the second youngest and myself. I can remember many times where I was told I couldn't hang out with my siblings because I was just a little kid or simply told to get away. They would tell me that only the big kids were hanging out. No matter what I did or said, I could not be a part of their group during those times. That feeling of not being accepted or part of the group makes you feel alone and sad. It is the same as children who form groups at school like the horse club, and only children who ride horses could be a part of the group.

This can happen at any time in our lives; it can even happen in adulthood. I moved to a new town once and was told by some moms that they already had enough friends. Those comments can make you feel like you don't belong. This sense of belonging and significance is part of human nature. It helps us find our place in the world and feel like we are a part of something.

In her book *The Gifts of Imperfection*, Brené Brown stated, "A deep sense of love and belonging is an irreducible need of all women, men and children."[10] She wrote that we will not function our best when we don't get that deep sense of love and belonging.[10]

So how do children experience or feel the love? It may not be as simple as "I love you," that gives us that genuine feeling of unconditional love. Years ago, I was part of a small group that studied a book by Gary Chapman and Ross Campbell called *The Five Love Languages of Children*.[11] It held the idea that we all, including children, experience the feeling of being loved in different ways. Some of us crave the words, or some of us long to be hugged. Others wish someone would spend time with them. Throughout the book, it identified that we are all wired in some way that makes us feel that innate sense of love. I learned through this study that I feel the most loved when someone does something kind for me. According to Chapman and Campbell, this is an act of service. The idea that someone would take time to do something just for me makes me feel special, and in that, I know that they care about me.[11]

When I had children and realized they weren't like me, I also learned that my children didn't feel love the same way I did. The way that they felt that connection or sense of belonging was different from the way that I did. As a parent, this can be challenging because it may be against our nature. My children would seek my attention in different ways, and I realized that they each had a unique love language. In their work on *The Five Love Languages of Children*, Chapman and Campbell highlighted five significant ways that children feel love.[11] This book clearly illustrated ways to incorporate this language into a child's life. Many children tend to have one language that is more dominant than others, although there can be more than one, which can change over time. If a caregiver or therapist understands how a child feels loved, you can create a bond and increase their sense of belonging and significance.

The five ways that children receive love, according to Chapman and Campbell,[11] are:

> Physical Touch
> Words of Affirmation
> Quality Time
> Gifts
> Acts of Service

At www.5lovelanguages.com, you can take a quiz to see what love language is your preference or a child's preference. These love languages are the same for adults, so as I go through them briefly, think about what makes you feel the most loved by those around you.

When a child's love language is *physical touch*, the sense of being close to an adult, a hand on their shoulder, a hug from a parent, tickle fights, and back scratches are all examples of physical touch. This feeling of physical contact makes them feel that they are safe and secure.[11]

My daughter, when she was little, always needed to be close to me. She craved hugs, snuggles, and no matter where we went, she would hold my hand. She would even reach for strangers' hands or climb on laps of friends when they came to visit just to be close to someone. If she were upset, you could see her body relax when she came for a hug. I didn't need to say anything to her. I would hug her, and she would be calm. She knew that she was okay and that she was loved. Her love language was physical touch.

A child can also feel loved through *words of affirmation*. This can be more than the words "I love you." It can be any "words of affection and endearment, words of praise and encouragement, words that give positive guidance" (p. 45).[11] The words should not be tied just to their actions; instead, it should be that they are loved for just who they are.

Children who have words of affirmation as their primary love language will beam when they hear the words like "It's so nice to see you," "You're awesome," "I love having you around," "You're doing great," or "You've got this," to name a few.

Quality time is when someone provides you with their undivided attention. This love language can be challenging in our busy lives. Real quality time is when you can be fully present with a child. Talking to them when you are cooking dinner or checking your phone is not quality time. Rather, it is creating time when you can look them in the eyes as you communicate together. You are present in your body language and your responses. You are putting away the devices that can distract you. Making time for one-on-one conversation and activities builds the connection that helps the child feel loved. Even attending sports events, doing errands together, or helping them with projects or work is quality time. It can be difficult when a child is part of a larger family, as they may never feel that they have that one-on-one time. Making sure to set aside time to fill their needs is vital for children who crave quality time.[11]

Children whose love language is *gifts* often feel that somebody loves them when they receive gifts. Many of us will get excited about a gift we receive, but to someone whose love language is gifts, the gift can represent the person's love for them. Have you ever seen a child who jumps up and down when they get a gift? They love the way it looks or feels, and when they open it, they get so excited. They are grateful for whatever they got. The gift brings them joy all day long, and when they ask who gave them that gift, they might respond, "My mom; she loves me." The idea that somebody thought of you and went out of their way to buy you something can make you feel special.[11]

Acts of service reflect the final love language that Chapman and Campbell touched on. This language is the one I described in the beginning as the way I feel loved. Have you ever had someone bring you tea when you hadn't asked for one? Or someone did a chore for you that you were supposed to do? These are examples of acts of service. Parents are always helping their children as they are growing up, but children who feel love through acts of service will note the times their parent or caregiver did something to help them. They may recognize love as when a parent helped with math homework, or a science project, or practiced shooting basketballs with them, or driving them to an important game.[11]

> *Thinking about the different ways of receiving love, what is your preference?*

Why is it important to understand a child's love language?

When we understand how children feel that they are loved, we can help them feel that they belong. Because if we don't think that we are loved, we tend to struggle with finding our place in the world and never reach our potential. A child's feeling of love does not just come from a parent or caregiver. The sense of love and belonging can come from anyone around them, including a teacher. The way a child feels connected to the people who are around them can affect the way they participate and experience that environment.

My mother-in-law was a grade school teacher. She taught in the primary grades for her whole career. Her ability to create a bond amongst her students was incredible to see. Years after her students were taught by her, they would return to tell her the impact that she had on them that year. Her students became a family. At the beginning of the year, the class would talk about how they wanted to be treated and what it meant to be a part of this group. Together, they would set the values of the class. Each child in the class felt that they were special to her. Every morning she would greet each child by name as they entered her classroom. For the kids, she was always fully present to listen to their stories. She shared words of encouragement. She would bring in small treats just to celebrate the class being who they were. She would allow children who needed to be near someone to sit next to her to work on school work. She created an atmosphere that covered all the different love languages. Each child felt the sense of love and belonging that one desires, even though their love languages were different.

We need to start by understanding our differences to understand how to make the environment inclusive and welcoming to everyone.

Our affective being goes beyond our sense of belonging and love. It goes into the way that our emotions respond to events that are going on around us. A child might laugh when they are scared or cry when they are happy. These emotional responses will differ from child to child. As adults, we need to be careful not to judge a child by their emotional response, as it may be the way they are wired. Some people laugh at a funeral. This doesn't mean it is funny; it can happen when we are nervous or uncomfortable. We never want to make assumptions based on how we would react; instead, we should have an element of curiosity to recognize what makes us unique.

Cognitive Being

A child can also be understood through the way that they think or learn. The way we process and understand information can be different for each of us. We may have different strengths that affect how we remember information based on our previous knowledge and experience.

Understanding how children learn is important for a child's growth and development, which we will dive into detail in a future chapter. The way a child learns impacts how they should be taught. A child's understanding of language can impact how they receive information. Have you ever told a joke in a room and some people didn't get it? This can be a difference in the way that a person interprets words. Taking the information that we learn through our different senses, our brain's ability to retain the information can be stronger for some children in one sense over the other.

Each component of a child that has been covered so far in this chapter outlines again how unique each person is. We are all physically different from one another; we think differently, and we feel differently. One is not better than the other; instead, the differences make this world an even more beautiful place. We should remain curious whenever we meet people in our goal to understand who they are and how they see the world.

Connection to the Caregiver

In the last chapter, we looked at the caregiver's connection and how it can affect the child. Who a child becomes or how a child behaves can be related directly to their caregiver.

Sarah was a four-year-old girl full of energy, who loved adventure, was occasionally a little loud, and would ask many questions. Her zest for life beamed from her. Her spirit of wonder and adventure was contagious—contagious only to those who recognized it and encouraged it.

Sarah was in an afterschool program at a neighbor's house. She would go straight from school to this home until her parents could pick her up. There were several children at this home, but none were as loud or energetic as Sarah. Anytime Sarah would get excited about something, she would talk loudly and jump up and down. This caregiver felt that Sarah needed to learn how to control her energy and constantly demanded that she stop or made her be by herself. Sarah realized that this caregiver didn't like who she was, and she would become upset when she had to go to the house after school because she didn't feel that she belonged. Each day when Sarah would get home from this afterschool program, all the emotions that she had bottled up would come out like a waterfall—to the point that her parents didn't know what happened. Sarah was unable to express what her feelings were, and she felt so unsettled in her skin.

Sarah's relationship with the caregiver in the afterschool program stifled her energy as a person. She was sensing that it wasn't right to be the way she was. This relationship changed how Sarah experienced that environment and, in the future, made her unsure of how she should act around others and if they would like her for who she was.

It is not only the way we as caregivers see children, but also the way a child senses the caregiver's feelings towards them that will impact how they respond and how they behave. If children feel loved and accepted for who they are, they are more likely to be open and expressive. If a child is fearful, then they will respond differently.

Just like Brené Brown wrote, the sense of love and belonging is a need of all humans, and if a child doesn't sense that from a caregiver in their life, they will struggle to find their place and reach their potential.[10]

Environment

Just like we had to understand the caregiver's environment, we also need to understand the environment as it relates to the child—the physical, institutional, social, and cultural elements.[4] What influences are affecting the child today? The environmental influences can impact a child's sense of belonging, connection, and safety.

When the physical elements match a child's needs, a child can feel more comfortable in that space. Just like the story of Johnny at the beginning of this chapter, the gymnastics class was more conducive to his learning than the classroom because of his ability to move. For some children, it may take them a while to feel comfortable in new environments. If a child is seen in a clinic setting, it may take a few visits for the child to get used to the physical space and feel comfortable to then build that trust with the therapist. It can be the same with school or groups outside of the home.

Children can be more relaxed when they are within their own home or space. There is comfort in some of the physical elements that belong to them. Think about a child who carries around a teddy bear or a blanket. It helps them have a sense of comfort. The comfort within the environment that the child is in may also affect how the child behaves. Often, children will let their guard down at home. That is a place that can provide comfort and safety for the child and allows their emotions to come out. This can be the opposite if the home is causing the challenges, and then a child may not find that a safe space and may hold their emotions in till they are at school.

Children can also be affected if something unpleasant or disturbing happened in an environment. For example, if a child witnessed or was in a car accident, the child may have a fear that may make them feel unsafe in the car. The same can happen in restaurants, planes, or trains or any place that makes a child feel unsafe. A child may display anxiety or avoidance behaviors when they are required to go to that space. The child may not be able to communicate their feelings, but they may have subconscious reactions and not know why.

Each physical space that a child interacts in often has institutional elements that include the rules and procedures required to be followed within each environment. School is an example with its own set of rules and expectations. These are more obvious to a child than rules set in the home setting. That is why children are often apprehensive, nervous, and anxious about the start of school. Having a new teacher and a new classroom environment will mean that they will have to get to know their teacher, other students, and a new set up. Their teacher will often develop their own set of class rules. It is often how a student can work within these rules and boundaries that can affect if they can "fit in" within this environment.

Religious buildings, government buildings, and medical buildings are other examples of physical spaces that have institutional elements that set the guidelines for behavior and expectations. For children, it can be hard for them to understand the different rules in regard to behavior. I experienced this with my children at the dentist office. They were going to a dentist who had an indoor play structure similar to the ones that they have at an indoor play park— climbing structures with tunnels and slides, with multiple levels. When children are at an indoor play park, they can be loud and yell to each other as they are moving around. At the dentist office, the expectations were a bit different, as they needed to remain relatively quiet while the staff were calling clients. If a child has difficulty understanding the rules of each environment, it may impact how they behave. For example, if a child never sits at home to eat a meal, it may be difficult for them to sit in a restaurant.

The social elements of an environment can also impact that feeling of belonging and safety. How a child is treated by teachers, therapists, parents, caregivers, family, and friends will impact how they feel in each situation.

When I was young, I remember going to one of my first sleepovers. I never really stayed overnight at many people's homes. We had no grandparents or cousins in town or even nearby. If we ever traveled, my parents would be with us. When I went to this sleepover, I distinctly remember being nervous, but excited. I didn't know what to expect. My mom had packed me red licorice to share with my friends when I got to the party. So, when we unpacked our things and set up for the night, I shared the licorice with all my friends. We left the room to play some more while we were eating our licorice. The girl's older sister was upset that she didn't have a licorice, but instead of asking for one, the mom called all the kids together to tell us a story. It was a story about a little girl who brought licorice to a sleepover and didn't share it with everyone, which made someone sad. I was five years old, and I was devastated. I was a pleasing child and never wanted anyone's feelings to be hurt or to feel sad. I hadn't even realized she was around when we were playing. I started crying and couldn't stop crying. My emotions had hijacked my brain, and all I knew was that I did not feel I belonged in this space and needed to go somewhere safe. I recall being picked up shortly after that. This event was so small, yet that moment affected my sense of safety in other people's homes for many years. The mom in this story, although unintentional, impacted my feeling of belonging.

Sometimes, this same experience can happen within the schools. Working as an occupational therapist in the classroom setting allowed me to see many different teacher–child interactions. I often would take a child out of the classroom to work on some skills in a quieter location. We didn't want to be a distraction to the rest of the class. In one particular class, when I knocked on the door to ask to see one of the children, the teacher's response was: "Sure, but it's not going to help anyway." I was as flabbergasted as you are reading this right now. The idea that a teacher would say this out loud in front of the class was horrific. What was even sadder was that this teacher did not believe in the child's potential. A child who hears that extra help won't make a difference is being inundated with messaging that does not encourage a child to try or even believe in themselves. Nor is this environment creating a sense of belonging.

How a child feels from the social elements of the space can impact their desire to stay within that environment. Would you want to stay somewhere where you knew you weren't wanted?

Think about this situation for a moment. A child is in a classroom setting where they are called out repeatedly for their behavior, or the class is so overwhelmingly loud, which causes them to act out. They have the feeling that they don't belong in their class. If the child craves a quiet space and feels a connection to the principal, being sent to the principal's office may be something that they want, as it helps them calm down.

Do you see how this could create a cycle of escape that could repeat itself? The child acts out, gets sent to the principal's office, finds calm, and returns to class.

What if a child was struggling in the classroom, and the teacher couldn't relate to the child, sends them to the principal, who also makes the child feel uncomfortable, where would that child go then?

This happened to another child I worked with. He was unable to find a space where he felt that he belonged and felt safe and secure while he was at school. He, therefore, became a flight risk from the school, and he would leave the school and run home. It became harder to get the child to return to school, as the child did not feel that he belonged.

Understanding how to connect with a child is one of the most important steps in building trust with a child.

The cultural elements of an environment can be intertwined in each of the previous elements. A religious building may have its own rules, but may also be influenced by a certain culture, such as a Polish Catholic Church. A family may have certain family traditions that are practiced within the home that will influence the activities that they can participate in, such as Shabbat dinners on Friday nights. Even family traditions and routines such as family games nights or holiday dinners can be examples of cultural elements that a child may participate in.

How to create an environment conducive to a child's learning is going to depend on their sense of belonging and love. This will also depend on how they process information through their sensory systems and how they learn. When you can understand these essential elements, you can create a space that makes children feel that they belong and are understood. In a future chapter, I will cover some specific environmental adaptations that can help a child once the caregiver has identified their unique sensory and learning needs.

Development

How children experience the world can also depend on a child's development. As children develop, there have been some consistencies that have been seen throughout all children. A child will often learn how to roll before they know how to crawl. A child will learn to stand before they walk. When the same development stages exist, it has created developmental milestones. These developmental milestones have set standards that many of the health care professionals follow. They give us a guideline for how a child will naturally progress through the developmental stages. Yet we need to remember that they are only guidelines.

And that is how it should stay—a guideline.

Guidelines can help us to flag some delays and direct our attention to building skills in different areas. We need to recognize that every child will develop at their own rate and to their own specific capabilities. The focus should be more on what those capabilities are and progressing those abilities.

The guidelines assist us to keep our eye on a target, but they should not be used alone. They should be used as a piece of the larger picture.

The child's physical, affective, and cognitive information will give us information about the child's abilities. The environment and the caregiver can also provide us with information about how a child is developing or will develop.

A child who is not crawling by 12 months would seem behind the general guidelines. What you need to look at is all parts of the child's story to understand why this child may be behind.

Does the child have the physical capacity to crawl?
Does the child have the cognitive ability to learn?
Does the child feel safe in this space?
Is the environment conducive to a child crawling?
Do those around the child encourage this progression?

I worked with a mom of a small child who was labeled "failure to thrive." The mom was struggling with postpartum depression and had not sought out care for herself. I am not sure how often her son was attended to, but she told me that he slept for 20 hours of the day on his back, and when he was awake, he would spend the rest of the time being held or in a recliner chair. The child had the physical capacity to crawl and learn, but he was not given the opportunity to learn. This can hinder the development of a child's skills. In this situation, helping the mother was integral in helping the child.

When a child enters school, they often have developed the finger grasps to hold a pencil or use scissors when they enter kindergarten or Grade 1. The ability to develop these skills can be dependent on the child's exposure to those skills. I received a referral for a child who could not hold a crayon or use scissors in Grade 1. The child's mother did not like her child to get messy or make a mess and, therefore, never let them play with crayons, use scissors, or even feed themselves. The caregiver and the environment affected the child's ability to learn the skills. The child was physically capable, but emotionally, they were so fearful of getting dirty that they were hesitant even to try.

Developmental milestones are important, but they need to be taken in the context of the child's entire story.

Be Careful With Labels

If a professional identifies that a child isn't developing at the same rate, expected capacity, or has some physical difference, they will sometimes give that child a diagnosis or a label. The two children who were behind in learning their skills may have a diagnosis of developmental delay, meaning that they are not developing at the same rate as the average child. Some more examples are a learning disability, which means that the child struggles with an area of learning. Physical disability means that their physical body does not function the same as the average person in some way. Sensory processing disorder means that they have difficulty processing the sensory world in a way that the average child processes it. Attention-deficit/hyperactivity disorder may mean a child has difficulty focusing amongst other factors.

A diagnosis or label can help us identify and communicate what challenges a child may have, but it doesn't tell us what their abilities are or what other factors are part of their story. For the two children we discussed in the last section, their delay in reaching the goals was in part from their exposure or care. The label of developmental delay does not highlight what potential reason they are behind. We need to make sure that a diagnosis or label never limits what a child can do.

Consider Nik Vujicic[8] at the beginning of this chapter, who was born with no arms or legs, which gave him a physical disability. His physical disability didn't tell us what he was capable of or what his full potential was.

Labeling a child who is not developing as expected can have both positive and negative impacts. When a child gets a diagnostic label, this can often help them to get the support they need or funding for services. They can get accommodations that may help them to be more successful. The challenge is that, sometimes, a label can change the expectations of the child. If a child is diagnosed with a learning disability, the expectations for how well they will do may be lowered. What is more important is understanding what they are capable of: how a child can learn the best rather than what they don't know.

I hear many stories about children who struggle in school, and they or their parents are told by people in positions, such as doctors, teachers, or guidance counsellors, that they should set their expectations lower in terms of life goals. These parents and children can believe less in their potential because of something someone told them. What if it was those limiting beliefs that were affecting their abilities? I have heard children say they are not going to try because they were told they'll never be good at something. This is a story that they continue to tell themselves.

When we are working with children, whether they are our own or a client, our job is to create opportunities to help them reach their potential and help them see a different story in themselves.

I have experienced the same challenges while working in the schools with children referred to me for behavioral concerns. They can be labelled as behavioral children. Yet, many times, I notice when I do my assessment that these children struggle with other aspects of learning, such as printing. There can be multiple reasons why this is happening, including eye–hand coordination or visual perceptual skills, but depending on their age, it can be challenging to teach them to print fast enough that it matches their ability to tell a story. Many of these children are so frustrated that they have behaviors and meltdowns when they are required to write. Their brain functions faster than their hands do. Yet many have an amazing story and a creative mind. The behavior is what becomes the focus at school, instead of what they are struggling with.

It again goes back to perspective. If the focus is on the behavior, you will miss the cause. If the focus is on the difficulty of printing, you will understand the behavior and can make accommodations. If the child has a diagnosis or label, we can use it as a clue, but not make it a limiting belief in the child's potential.

Throughout this chapter, we have covered many different points that can impact how a child engages: from the way that they feel loved to the different environmental elements that they are exposed to, to the way a child develops and the labels a child is given. Each of these areas gives us clues into a child's story. It encourages us to ask questions and stay curious.

As you continue to progress through this book, I will try to engage your curiosity into other characteristics of how a child engages in the world, starting with the sensory system.

Chapter Reflections

1. Why is it important to look at the abilities of a child instead of disabilities?
2. What does love languages mean?
3. What are the five love languages?
4. Why should we look at developmental milestones as guidelines?
5. What are the benefits and risks with labelling a child?

5   Acknowledging the Sensory World

One of the keys to unlocking part of a child's story is understanding how they experience the physical world. How does the brain interpret sensory experiences? Each of our physical bodies is created with a sensory system that sends signals to the brain. The brain processes the information. What the brain then tells the body about that information will be different for each person.

The sensory system is made up of eight different sensory inputs. The first five familiar to us include touch, smell, taste, vision, and hearing. The three that we don't often think about, but are essential to our everyday functioning, are the vestibular, proprioceptive, and interoception systems. Each of the systems can be assessed by asking the following questions:

What does this sensory system tell us?
What are the common challenges?
What are examples of dysfunction?
What does this mean?

When one sensory system is under- or over-functioning, it will change how a child responds in different environments. Research has been done to understand how we process sensory information, understand how the senses work together, or identify deficits that might exist. In the rest of this chapter, I will highlight an overview of the systems.

Understanding how a child reacts to and experiences the world through their senses will help us gain clues into what makes them who they are and how we can help them navigate the complexities in the world.

So, What Is the Sensory World?

Have you ever walked into a room, and it felt like home? Or walked into a space that reminded you of your childhood?

For me, it was the smell of muffins cooking in the oven or the smell of my dad's aftershave before he went to work.

DOI: 10.4324/9781003166405-5

The sensory world is how we experience all aspects of the world: the world we see, hear, touch, smell, taste, and move around in. The sensory world is ever changing, and no two people will experience the world the same.

We often forget about how much our sensory system has gotten used to the world around us. Think about a baby touching water for the first time and the quick reaction to avoid the touch of the water, as it is a new experience. Now think for a moment about the last time you touched water, whether it was washing your hands or it was taking a shower. You may not have even thought twice before you put your hands or feet in the water.

Think about the smell of a summer rainfall, or the sound of birds chirping in their nest, or when you saw your first rainbow. Think now about the clothes that you wear. The way your pants feel against your legs, or the shirt rubbing across your chest, or the underwear around your waist. We have become so accustomed to some of the sensory inputs in the environment or to our body that we don't sense them anymore. How often do you think about your pants rubbing against your legs? How often do you walk outside and not hear the birds chirping? If you can say that you hardly notice them anymore, you have developed an excellent ability to regulate your sensory inputs.

Our body has many ways to receive information from all around us to help us navigate the world. These inputs feed into our one control center, also known as our brain, and this is where we process that information. Our brain stores and categorizes what we have experienced so that when we experience it again, our brain can recognize and react. Our brain will also let us know if this is an okay situation or if we should be alarmed.

For some people, their brain recognizes many inputs as alarming. Some can't tolerate clothes brushing against their legs because it feels like sandpaper. Some can't stand the sound of crying because it sounds like owls screeching. If the connection to the brain sends the wrong signal or can't find where the information is stored, we may have reactions that are not consistent with the input.

I am sensitive to noise. I have been since I was little. If there is a ticking clock in a room, that is the only sound I can hear despite my strongest desire to concentrate on something else. All I can hear is the ticking.

Tick. Tick. Tick. Tick.

I have been in exams and unable to finish because of ticking clocks, or someone chewing gum, or someone tapping their pencil. The overwhelming input from sensory inputs in a brain can hijack your ability to disregard that information and focus on something else.

If our body does not tolerate the inputs, our brain will send a signal that tells the rest of the systems in the body that "This information is not okay." We need to fight it, put up a resistance, run away from it, or withdraw from the situation—also known as our fight-or-flight response.

Our processing of the sensory world is so instantaneous that, for the most part, many of us hardly even recognize its existence; for others, it can challenge their everyday functioning.

Your Sensory Preferences

If you are reading this book, chances are you have been around for at least a few years and have developed your sensory preferences. Sensory preferences are the activities that you have decided you enjoy doing and the things that you avoid.

A good example is if you think for a moment about the very last thing you do before you go to sleep.

When you are getting ready for bed, what do you need to do before going to sleep?

I have done this activity with moms in different groups, and the answers I get are always so diverse.

Some need to have some tea right before bed.
Some need to have a sound machine on.
Some need the room cold, others warm.
Some need a heavy comforter, and some require a light comforter.
Some wear socks, and some wear nothing at all.
Some need to scroll on their phone.

We all have developed a sense of when we feel the calmest. When we get to this feeling, our body can almost breathe a sigh of relief.

It is similar to when you start your day. You may have the same routine every day that helps you get your day started just the way you like it.

Breakfast. No breakfast.
Coffee. Tea.
Socks. No socks.
Music in the background. News.

Whatever your routine is, it came to be because of your sensory preferences. How you greet the day sets up your body for a sense of calm. If you don't start the day the way you like it, this can lead to a sense of unrest. Similar to going to bed. We fall asleep when we can find our sense of calm.

These sensory preferences have developed over time. We often don't recognize how much we have in place until something changes, and we feel out of sorts.

We need to be really aware of how long it has taken us to get to the point we are now; we must understand that children are still trying to figure it all out. They are trying to understand what feels right and what doesn't. If a child's communication has not developed enough to identify what isn't feeling right, they may react with different behaviors, anxiety, or fear.

This is why it is crucial to understand what makes up our sensory system. This knowledge helps us to understand what elements in the child's environment might be impacting how they behave. How does sensory information get processed in the brain, and how do our bodies interpret it? How can we help children find their preferences?

Sensory Systems

Our sensory system is made up of eight different systems. Each one provides information to the brain that helps our bodies understand and navigate the world. Because they are housed in one body, the systems all work in conjunction with each other. For example, we often see what we are touching, so our brains can prepare our minds for what we feel. If we see a tree, we would expect it to be rough when we touch it. If we smell cookies baking, we would expect to taste the cookies when we eat them. When we walk in a forest, our vision helps our body prepare for uneven ground, and our touch receptors help us find a solid footing while smelling the moss and pine around us.

---

8 Sensory Systems

Touch
Smell
Taste
Visual
Hearing
Vestibular
Proprioception
Interoception

By understanding each system's purpose, you can then see how limitations in that system or systems can affect how a child engages in a specific environment or with people. When we are exposed to all the varied sensory inputs, our bodies decide what we do with this information. If our brain finds the sensory input pleasurable, we will have a positive response to it. Suppose our brain, on the other hand, does not find the information enjoyable. In that case, we may have a more unpleasurable response, such as a fight-or-flight response as described earlier, which tells us to either defend ourselves or find safety.

This response can happen when people experience a sensory input that is not desirable, or their ability to process what is going on leaves them feeling so overwhelmed.

Liam was in Grade 2 when I saw him. He had difficulty with verbal communication, both receiving it and expressing it. It meant that he had trouble understanding any spoken words and could only say a few words himself. When the classroom environment became loud with lots of people talking, and then the teacher tried to speak over the top of everyone else's voice, Liam found the input overwhelming. On occasion, Liam would become agitated and push his chair or desk; other times, Liam walked out of the classroom. His body had gone into the fight-or-flight response, and he needed to react to get himself to a safe space. As a therapist working with Liam, we first had to identify what brings him to this state by understanding how he processes the sensory information. Once we understood his triggers or activities that irritated him, we could then work on strategies to help him find calm or a just-right state. The goal would be to eventually get Liam to regulate his own needs, which I will cover in Chapter 7.

As we look at all the different sensory systems, think about how you process this type of information. Then try to think about those around you. How have you seen these sensory preferences or sensitivities expressed by others around you, especially the children you work with?

Touch

We have thousands and thousands of nerve endings around our entire body that send signals to our brains about what we are feeling. This is our sense of touch. We can feel the sensation all over our skin as well as in our mouths, throat, and ears. Did you know we even have touch receptors inside our bodies, in our stomach and around our organs? The sense of touch is our first sensory system to develop and develops as we grow inside our mother's uterus. It is also the largest sensory system out of all of them and provides a lot of input to our brain through two different pathways.[12] Our touch receptors can even distinguish between light and deep pressure, hot and cold, and pain.[13] This is important because the way that our body will respond to touch receptors will differ.

Imagine you were sitting on the grass reading a book. You can feel the firmness of the ground beneath you. You can feel the blades of grass on your feet. Then as you are sitting there, you sense the light rhythmic sensation moving up your leg. That sensation is unlike the feeling of the grass or the ground. Your brain is triggered to alert you of this unusual sensation, and you often move or swat at your leg. You then can see that the feeling on your leg was a spider crawling up your leg. This very light touch can trigger an unpleasant reaction. I'm sure many of us shiver even thinking about this.

When my daughter was little, she hated any pants that were not tight to her leg. The texture of jeans or corduroy would put her into fits of screaming till the pants were removed. It was the light brushing of the material on her legs that she couldn't tolerate.

Our light-touch receptors can be activated by the brushing of a shirt on your body, the wind passing by, someone walking too close, underwear, or socks on the feet. It can also be activated by someone breathing too closely or the fabric on a chair. If you are sensitive to light touch, it can be the faintest of feelings that can elicit a response.

The opposite of light touch is when you experience deep pressure. Think of the feeling of a child running up to you and giving you a great big bear hug.

The tight squeeze around your neck triggers the deep pressure receptors, which feed a different signal to your brain. The same can be said for that feeling when you lie under a heavy blanket or when you sit on a soft couch or bean bag chair. I have had children at school who craved deep pressure throughout the day, as it helps them feel calm and would reset their sensory system.

The two different ways our body interprets touch can be divided into protective and discriminatory.[12] The signal travels to the brain in two different pathways. The protective sensation quickly alerts your brain if there is danger, such as something is hot. It then allows you to respond rapidly by telling your body to move. The discriminatory sensation sends a signal to your brain to give it information about what you are touching, such as the shape, texture, or size. At this point in your life, you may be able to put your hand in a bag and find your cell phone without looking or reaching for your car keys.[12] Sometimes, our protective sensations can be heightened and may react to many inputs as being dangerous even when they are not.

The touch receptors in our mouths are often more complex, as the texture and temperature of food are dynamic. Within our mouths, we also have our gustatory or taste buds, olfactory or smell, and our vision of the food that can affect how and what we eat.

When it comes to texture aversions, my son struggled with this when he was little. He loved to eat yogurt, but he could not handle the texture of chunks in his yogurt. Anytime there were chunks, it would cause him to gag. The yogurt's taste was not the issue, as he loved flavored yogurt, but it was the consistency that bothered him. Whenever he was fed yogurt, he would gag and spit up what he had eaten. The daycare that he was at would often call us to come and get him, as they would say that he was sick to his stomach. Not even realizing the cause and effect at the time, it took us a while to understand that his body responded to the chunks in the yogurt as a threat, and it would make him gag and spit it out. To this day, he still despises any food he eats that has chunks in it.

Think for yourself, have you ever poured yourself a glass of milk, and when you went to drink it, it had curdled and had chunks in. Because you expected to have smooth milk, your brain alerted you that there were chunks in the milk, and you spit it out.

It's your body's way of protecting itself from a threat. A child might interpret food as a threat because of texture, taste, or smell. This could create the response that their body wants them to get to a safe space, which may be spitting food out.

Our sense of touch is continuously giving us clues about the world around us. Think about the feeling of this book as you read it. Whether it is on a tablet or paper; what does it feel like? What does the chair feel like where you are sitting or the clothes that you are wearing? Your awareness of these sensory inputs will help you investigate and acknowledge the way a child feels. For example, look at their clothing preferences, if they like big hugs or light back tickles, or if they tend to sit very close or avoid any contact.

According to Biel and Peske,[12] tactile defensiveness is one of the most well-known sensory challenges. When someone is defensive to any touch input, they are hypersensitive to that feeling and react negatively or withdraw from that input. This defensiveness can range from mild to severe. Mild defensiveness could be when you don't like a particular texture on your skin or when someone brushes past you, such as a child waiting in a class line. An extreme version is when the touch sends you into a panic, such as if someone puts their arm on you. The opposite of being defensive is being under-sensitive. A child who doesn't react when they have been hurt or seeks out deep input, wanting to play wrestle or be wrapped tight in blankets, may be under-sensitive to the signals coming in.[12]

Smell

Also known as olfactory, our sense of smell is one of our primitive senses. Think about what happens when you smell something that you had in your childhood? The scent of a certain meal, a particular cologne, or the smell of your clean laundry can remind you of moments in your past. Specific memories will be triggered by our sense of smell, whether good or bad. We use this sense to inform us about the environment we are in. It can warn us if something isn't right. We can smell gas in the air, smoke, or rotten food, which tells us to avoid something or get help. If your sense of smell is hypersensitive, it can create a noxious or unpleasant response to a minimal amount of scent in the air.

Think for a moment about your space right now.

What do you smell?

Now, think about a school classroom during lunch break, or a gymnasium with sweaty Grade 8 students, or the smell of car exhaust, or the diesel of a bus and how overwhelming these daily smells might be for a child. Even the smell of food cooking may trigger an adverse reaction. People who are hypersensitive to smells can walk around, always feeling overwhelmed by the world around them. The opposite is someone who has an under-sensitive response. This would be someone who hardly notices the smells around them. They may not be able to smell flowers or rotten food, and they may crave more input to create any reaction.[12]

My son is sensitive to smells. The smell of something cooking can trigger a response that makes him upset or excited about dinner. If the smells trigger an unpleasant memory, even if it is not the same food being cooked, he will put up a fight to even get to the table. If the smell is familiar and he has a good memory of it, he will come to the table without a fight.

Because smells can trigger memories, it can also remind you of a time or place that was pleasant for you and can create a reaction in your body that makes you feel calm. I will discuss how our senses can play into our ability to calm ourselves in Chapter 8.

Our sense of smell is also a critical component of our sense of taste.

Taste

Our sense of taste or gustatory sense is how our brain identifies the food we eat. We only have five different types of taste buds. We have a sense of sweet, sour, bitter, salty, and umami. These receptors are in various areas of our tongue. The sense of taste works with the sense of smell to give us the pleasurable or non-pleasurable responses to food.

> *What happens to your favorite food when you plug your nose and try to eat it?*

It won't "taste" the same. When we discuss the tastes of food, it is hard to separate the two senses. Like the way our body reacts to smell, we can be hypersensitive to particular tastes, and our body can have a negative or positive response to it. Or our body can be under-sensitive to taste, and we have little to no reaction to different tastes.

Andrew was a premature baby. He was fed through a tube directly to his stomach till he was almost two years old. When he started learning how to take in food by mouth, he had developed extreme aversions to the texture of food, and his ability to taste food was limited. To help Andrew develop his brain's connection to his taste receptors, Andrew spent time with his occupational therapist to develop his taste receptors by exposing them to the five specific tastes. Trying to connect the brain's ability to recognize the taste, combined with the smell and the tolerance of textures, is needed to experience the food we eat. Although he was much better as he aged, Andrew would crave extra hot sauce on most of the foods to stimulate an increased sense of taste.

Visual

Our visual system or the way we see the world is more complicated than just looking at art pieces. The images that our eyes see are processed in our brain, and then our brain has to interpret the image and match it to a database of images. Then it identifies what we are seeing and lets the rest of our body know how to respond to what we see. For example, if we are watching a soccer game and the ball is heading straight for us, our brain has to process the ball's location and speed, then tell our body what to do with this information, such as move out of the way. Our brain doesn't just process the data from one visual input; for people with two working eyes, our brain has to take the information from two images and match them and then process what this means. Since our world is continuously moving and changing, our visual system is always at work. Do you ever wonder why your eyes feel tired at the end of the day? They have been working non-stop since the moment you woke up.

The visual system is extremely complex. There are so many parts that need to work together to see and understand a clear picture. For example, the system relies on the coordination of the muscles around our eyes to help our eyes move and focus. The shape of our eyeballs determines how our eyes process the light coming into our brain. Because the visual system is so complicated, there can be many different challenges impacting the information that our brain receives. If a child struggles with their visual processing, it is essential to check to make sure their visual system's physical components are working as they should.

I worked with Brian, a child in Grade 8 who was struggling to get his work done. His teacher felt he needed help with time management and organization. When I started working with him, I wanted to get a sense of where he was regarding his ability to process visual information. We started with the basics so that we could see what level he would get to. What surprised me is that he could not recognize individual letters of the alphabet, and it was not caught before this time. Our brain's ability to process letters and organize information is not innate; it is something that we have to be taught. Think about every written language around the world. The way it is written is different depending on who invented it. What we see on paper needs to be processed by our visual input into a catalog in our brains that identifies the shape and then matches it with the sound to describe the letter. It is a complex process that one in five children struggles with doing. When our brains can't process this, one diagnosis could be dyslexia.[14]

The brain's ability to process information will affect our body's response to what we see. If our two eyes cannot focus the same, we may feel a little off balance when we walk. Alternatively, if too much information is coming in simultaneously, such as walking in a crowd of people, our eyes may not know where to focus, and our brain may feel overwhelmed.

Visual stimuli can signal to the body a positive or negative emotional response, depending on how your brain processes information.

Think about how you feel when you look out over a body of water.
Think about how you feel when you look at a garbage dump.
Think about how you feel in a clean and tidy room.
Think about how you feel when you look at a messy kitchen.

The emotions that images can conjure within us show us how we need to be aware of what children see and how they react to it.

Have you ever been on a spinning ride at an amusement park? In our town, they call it The Scrambler. It is a ride where you are sitting in a small car, and when the ride starts, the car spins, and the arm it is attached to spins, and as the speed picks up, you spin faster and faster. It is hard for your eyes to focus on anything. That is because the information from our visual system is trying to send a signal to our brain, but our brain can't process the information fast enough, so the images are not very clear.

That is what being oversensitive may look like for a child who has difficulty processing visual information. It may not be fast moving like a ride, but a child staring at a classroom wall that is covered in bright-colored charts and words and pictures may have too much information coming in so that the brain can't process it. A child can have the same reaction if there are flashing lights at a hockey game or a school dance. When a child is overstimulated, you may see them close their eyes or stare at less overwhelming spaces. If a child is under-sensitive to visual inputs, you may see a child crave fast visual stimuli, such as video games, movies, and bright flashing lights.

Our visual system provides information about the food we are going to eat, the sounds we hear, how our body needs to move, and what we smell. It helps to unlock the responses that we need and how we should react. When this system is not working well, it can have a ripple effect into many other systems.

Hearing

What we hear is also known as our auditory sense. When we hear something in the world, it creates a vibration that makes waves that travel to our ears. The sound waves vibrate our eardrums, and the information is sent to our brains. Our brain, just like the catalog for our vision, has a record for all the different vibrations it needs to interpret.

Listen to the sounds you hear right now.

As I write this, I can hear the fan of the furnace in the background. I can hear the hum of the light above my computer, and I can hear my fingers typing on the keyboard. Most movements make a sound, and the environment those sounds are in will affect the sound waves' pattern. Think about the echo you hear in a tiled bathroom versus the dampening sounds in a carpeted room.

Our brain has to have the ability to process a sound and identify what a sound is. It also needs to interpret which sounds are most important to focus on, where the sound is coming from, and what the sound means. Since it is made up of many physical components, if a child is having difficulty with sound, it is always important to first make sure there is a good physical connection from the ear to the brain.

With the hearing system's complexity, it is not surprising to know that many students struggle to process auditory information. If a child can't process what a sound is or what it means, they may not have the appropriate reactions. Some children may be oversensitive to sounds and feel overwhelmed and anxious with certain noises. Some people can hear sounds that others don't hear, or they may experience every loud sound or certain decibels of sounds as a threat like a fire alarm, even if it is just the ringing of a telephone, a parent yelling, or the school lunch bell.

My son struggles with auditory processing. We noticed that he would not respond when we called him to come to the dinner table, especially when he was watching TV. He was overwhelmed when we had people at our house, and he would have difficulty recalling information he heard at school. Through an auditory processing assessment, we learned that his brain has a problem focusing when there are any competing sounds. It now made sense why he couldn't recall information from school because if someone were talking closer to him, he would have difficulty hearing what his teacher was saying. He was missing instructions and information about what to do in class and was feeling lost. It also made sense when we had people over. If too many people were talking simultaneously, he had trouble listening to any of them. Being aware of his challenges gave us information to help him make changes to support his environmental needs. I have worked with many children who struggle with similar challenges in processing auditory information.

Our auditory system works in conjunction with many of our other systems. One that it works closely with is our movement system. Have you ever wondered why when a baby hears a loud bang, they startle, or when you hear your favorite sound on the radio, you have that urge to move? Our auditory and vestibular system's receptors are located right next to each other and are connected within the inner ear. This is why when we hear something, it usually makes us react by moving.[12]

Vestibular

The vestibular system is our movement processing system. It tells us where our body is in space in relation to gravity. Since we are continually navigating against gravity, it is a system that is always working. Our vestibular system is located in our inner ear and tells us what the rest of our body needs to do to maintain our position in space. For example, if we reach down to pick something off the floor, our vestibular system sends a signal to our brain to tell specific muscles to activate so that we don't fall over. It is an instant reaction, and we don't even realize it is happening. Children who have difficulties with their vestibular system may not get that same quick reaction from their brains, so they may feel like they will fall or do fall when they reach down. The vestibular system also tells us if we are spinning, accelerating, or decelerating when we move. Think about when you are driving a car. When you first accelerate, you can feel that you are going faster, but your body doesn't feel the movement as much when you are going at the same speed. Likewise, when you decelerate.[12]

Working with children, I have seen several children who struggle with vestibular challenges and are hypersensitive or fearful of swinging, playing sports, or climbing on jungle gyms. They tend to fall a lot and are much more timid. Children with an extreme emotional response tied to any movement against gravity are referred to as having gravitational insecurity. They fear being pushed into movements or having their feet off the ground and are most settled when they sit on the floor. Children who are hyposensitive to the sensory inputs tend to crave movement opportunities. You will see these children gravitate towards swings, monkey bars, jumping on couches, or spinning, or even unique sitting positions, such as watching television upside down.[12]

Proprioception

Proprioception is your brain's ability to know where your body is in relation to itself. If you close your eyes, do you know where your hand is or where your feet are. This internal sensory system takes information from our nerves, ligaments, tendons, and joints and tells us where they are and need to be. For instance, when you take a spoonful of soup, you don't think about where your hand is and how it will get to your mouth. For many of us, this happens without us thinking about it anymore. Likewise, when we sit at a desk or a chair, we don't have to think about activating our muscles to keep us balanced and upright.

For children who struggle with proprioception, the lack of awareness of where their body is in space or the lack of feedback from their ligaments, tendons, and muscles can make it hard to do ordinary tasks. Children who struggle with fine motor activities, such as holding a pencil or doing up zippers and buttons, may have difficulty with proprioception. They may not feel the weight of the pencil or where the buttons are in relation to each other, and they tend to look clumsy or uncoordinated.

Jane was a girl I worked with who was referred to me for poor printing. She had difficulty holding her pencil because she couldn't sense the pressure that she was having on the pencil. To increase her body's ability to feel the pencil and react to it, we increased the pencil's weight. Her body was then able to create a reaction to counter the weight, which increased her ability to grip the pencil and control it.

Interoception

Interoception is the sensory system that we often don't think about. Have you ever thought about what gives you that urge to go to the washroom, or what gives you that urge to get yourself something to drink? That is called interoception. Our body is made up of many systems that keep our body functioning the way that it should. Our brain, heart, lungs, and digestive system all function without us thinking of them, but when we get scared and feel our heart race, it lets us know that we need to do something to get us back to the sense of safety or normalcy.

Children can struggle with interoception if they aren't aware of what their body is telling them. They may not get the urgent signals to use the washroom or confuse the signal with feeling afraid. Since their body sends them signals to help it stay functioning at a balanced state, if the signal is confused, it may lead to a stress response, including anxiety and fear.

Have you ever seen a child who gets angry when they need to use the washroom? Or children who have what we call "hangry" symptoms? Their bodies tell them they need to eat something, but they do not recognize the signal and instead act out. Before you treat the interoception as a sensory concern, it is always good to check with a doctor to ensure that all the systems are working okay first.[12]

Sensory Processing

How does our body take in all of these sensory inputs, and what does it do with them?

Each of our sensory systems plays a vital role in helping us navigate and experience the world. Yet each of our sensory systems and how they process information will be unique to the individual. That is what is key to understanding the children we work with. Although each system is different, they are integrated and often function together.

The way we take the information that we get from our sensory inputs and use or react to it is known as *sensory processing*. When the reactions are different than what is expected or a child is over- or under-reactive to a specific input, they may be having difficulties processing one or many sensory inputs. This can be referred to as sensory processing disorder.

Our brain also learns about sensory inputs and how to process them from exposure to sensory information. A child who was never allowed to climb on jungle gyms may have more of a fear reaction when their vestibular system experiences new positions, or a child who has never walked barefoot in the grass or felt sand on their feet may be fearful when they are exposed to these environments. These sensations may be overwhelming to a child, as the brain needs to process and categorize them. In some cases, controlled exposure to sensory input can help our brain build the pathways to recognize the sensation and have a neutral response to it.

Think about a child who is afraid of a washroom. Have you ever walked into a bathroom and thought about all the sounds, smells, textures, and movements you need to do in the bathroom? Children who are sensitive to sounds may be overwhelmed and fearful of the water's sound in the tap, the flushing of the toilet, or in a school washroom, the sound of the hand dryer. Just the sounds alone can be overwhelming to a child, then add in all the rest of the sensory experiences. A child may not be going to the washroom because of the sensory overload that using the bathroom brings.

Sensory overload is when your body receives so much sensory input that it cannot tolerate any more, and the person often tries to find ways to remove themself from that situation. A child throwing a tantrum when they have to use the bathroom can result from a sensory overload. A child who zones out during class because they no longer can focus on the teacher, copy work onto a paper, and focus on sitting simultaneously can be experiencing sensory overload. Sensory overload can look like negative behaviors to those who aren't aware of a child's sensory needs. The action that is usually exhibited is a *sensory avoiding* behavior: a child's way of avoiding whatever is making them uncomfortable.

If a child is under-responsive, meaning that it takes more input than average to activate that sensory system, a child may seek sensory input. For example, if a child needs a lot of movement to stimulate their vestibular system, they may be jumping from couch to couch or doing somersaults in the living room. It is known as *sensory-seeking* behavior.

When children seek or avoid sensory input, they are trying to get their bodies to that point of feeling just right or balanced. It is like the feeling of having a pebble in your shoe, and you are uncomfortable until you can get it out, then it all feels okay again.

Finding that "just right" feeling in one's sensory system is what we strive for with children. The challenge is that children often can't communicate what they need or what they don't like. Instead, what they will experience are meltdowns, behaviors, or withdrawal from situations.

A child's *sensory preferences* describe how a child's sensory system reacts in different situations. These can be compiled in a document that can be shared with others who are working with the child so that they can understand why the child may respond in certain situations and how to set up an environment that meets their needs. In their book, *Raising a Sensory Smart Child*, Biel and Peske[12] go into detail about a child's sensory needs. They also published a free checklist that goes through questions in every sensory category that will help you identify your child's preferences by how they react in different situations. This information and checklist can be found at: www.sensorysmartparent.com/checklist

Sensory Therapy

When children have difficulty processing sensory information, they can have trouble completing the activities they want or need to do. They may have difficulty focusing in class or tolerating the environment. Over the years, various theories and ideas have been developed that help children learn strategies to increase their independence and function.

A. Jean Ayres created one method. She developed the Ayres Sensory Integration® method, which uses a specific series of sensory constructs to help increase a child's ability to process sensory information. The idea is that our brains have neuroplasticity and can develop or change over time.[15]

Sensory diets or *sensory schedules* became more common as therapists came to understand the need to provide breaks throughout the day to meet a child's sensory needs. A sensory diet or schedule is a series of activities specific to the child, which breaks up the day and allows opportunities for the sensory input that they crave or need in order to find their balance. When you get a child to a balanced or "just right" state, as I referred to it earlier, the child may be able to engage in the classroom activity more effectively than if they were in an over- or under-responsive state.

The terms *sensory toys* have also become more popular as therapists discovered that certain toys could give a child the sensory input they crave and can either calm a child or increase their energy. A sensory toy may be something that has lights, sounds, vibrates, smells, or is soft or squishy. It will be dependent on the child's sensory preferences as to what activities they will gravitate towards.

When children are in a classroom, it is often difficult for them to move around and get their energy out. Some children would benefit from small squishy toys or little twisting toys that they could move in their hands. When a child was able to expend a little bit of their energy with even a small fidget, they would often find it increased their ability to listen and focus.

Understanding Our Differences

The child, caregiver, and our own sensory preferences will impact how we engage in activities throughout the day. An activity that may be calming for you or enjoyable may not be pleasant for the child and vice versa. Taking the time to learn about a child's sensory needs, similar to understanding their love language as discussed in the previous chapter, is a tool to discover what makes a child unique. In the next chapter, I will focus on how children learn new information and how this can impact their needs.

Chapter Reflections

1. What eight sensory systems help us experience the world?
2. What is the difference between over- and under-stimulation?
3. What is sensory processing?
4. What does it mean to have sensory overload?
5. Why is it important to understand a child's sensory preferences?

6 Understanding How Children Learn

When we only know part of a child's story, we can only make some guesses about all of the other aspects. This often leads to a child being misunderstood by their actions. One big factor is in knowing how children receive or process information. Understanding how children learn is complicated, just like it is to understand our sensory system. We can sometimes forget that others don't think or process information the same way we do, and we can get frustrated when a child doesn't "get it." Working with children, I have learned that recognizing the ways children learn is an essential piece to include in their story. It is not about IQ or specific learning difficulties; instead, it is about creating a supportive environment to help children learn. It includes how they use their sensory system to process information, understand language, match information to previous knowledge, their mindset, and what motivates them to learn. This chapter is intended to guide you through looking at the big picture when describing a child's learning needs.

The way a child processes information describes their cognitive or thinking abilities.[3] In this chapter, I explain what we do with the information we receive from our sensory systems discussed in the last chapter. Learning how much information our sensory system processes throughout the day, it is surprising how we make it through each day without feeling overwhelmed by all that we encounter.

Many of us have become so used to all the inputs we receive daily that we don't even notice a lot of what we see, feel, hear, smell, or touch unless we are mindful of it. Our bodies have learned how to only alert us to unusual or different inputs than our usual. This is not true for everyone. For some people, the body continues to react to alert them to inputs that happen every day, making it hard to function in their daily lives. Learning how to regulate our sensory information as well as our emotions will be covered in Chapter 8. Understanding how our sensory inputs can help us learn or affect how we receive and process new information is essential for understanding how kids learn.

Julie was a little girl I worked with who had difficulty processing all the sounds going on around her. Due to her auditory processing challenges, her ability to focus on a sound was difficult, especially if more than one person

DOI: 10.4324/9781003166405-6

or object was making noise. Her auditory memory was limited, which meant that she was unable to remember things she heard. In class, if she were given three- or four-step instructions, she wouldn't be able to follow them. For example, if she was in class, and the teacher said, "Sit down, take out your math notebook, turn to page 63, and begin looking at question four," she would be lost.

Julie was referred to occupational therapy to help with attention and focus. Julie always seemed to be lost in class, according to the teacher. When I worked with Julie, she described the feeling of not knowing what was going on. She said she also had the feeling of being lost or unsure what to do when she was at home and would usually stay in her room so that she wouldn't get asked to do anything by her mom.

In class, Julie felt like she missed some of the teacher's instructions and would have to look around to get an idea of what she was supposed to do. Julie was trying to use a lot of the environmental cues around her, looking at others, and watching what they did. Sometimes, she would get to the right spot on time, but other times, her teacher would catch her just sitting there waiting to be told again. When working with Julie, I noticed that her ability to follow instructions was limited. She was only able to follow two-step instructions. I also noticed that she would have difficulty maintaining focus on the instructions if there were any background noises. The challenge in a classroom setting with 25 other students is that there was always some background noise, and Julie didn't feel comfortable raising her hand to ask what they were supposed to do. Instead, she would slump in her chair and hope her teacher didn't notice her. By learning about Julie's needs, I communicated with the teacher what would help Julie stay on task. A specific change that was suggested related to how the teacher gave instructions. The teacher would say her instructions and then write them on the board so that Julie could look up and know what she was supposed to do. It made a considerable difference to Julie's ability to stay on task in class. I was also able to communicate with Julie's parents to understand how to engage Julie in activities at home by using a whiteboard or giving her written instructions.

This little change in communication helped Julie not only to be able to function more effectively in class, but also to decrease her stress and anxiety. Julie had felt lost, but didn't know why. She didn't realize that she wasn't hearing the teacher's instructions, yet she also didn't understand why everyone else knew what to do. Instead, she just felt overwhelmed in class. She was frustrated with herself and felt that her teacher was always upset with her. Taking the time to learn what makes Julie unique helped her be able to engage and participate in class again, confidently.

There are many Julies in the world who struggle to stay connected in class and often feel lost. Recognizing how a child processes information from the world around them will affect how they will best receive information, which can unlock a child's potential.

Learning Strengths

There are four different ways that we generally receive information. The first is through hearing information, which is known as auditory learning. The second is visual learning or through what we see. The third is tactile learning or when we can touch and feel objects, and the last is kinesthetic, which is learning through movement. These different ways of receiving information help us to learn about the world. Each of these ways includes our various senses, and each one plays a role in creating the memory.

Think about a flower. If I tell you about a rose and describe its features, you would develop a picture in your head of what a rose looks like. Yet that picture may be different for all of us. If I were to show you a picture, you would create a memory that pairs the information about the rose with the image, but the picture would still not explain what the rose smells like or what the rose feels like. To understand what a rose is, we need to experience the rose through all our senses and store it in our different memory files to recall what a rose is the next time we come across one.

Many of us may think that there is one way you prefer to learn, and that is something I always believed in as well. In their article "The Myth of Learning Styles," Riener and Willingham[16] summarized that research has not proven that we only learn through one way or that one way is stronger than another. Instead, what is more valuable to understand is someone's abilities, interests, and existing knowledge, which will affect how they process information. Using this information, you can then create learning opportunities that match this information. This can relate to how well a person retains and understands information, which will develop stronger connections in their brain.[16]

Our sensory system was covered in the last chapter. Each of us has different sensory preferences or ways that we process sensory information. For those who have difficulty focusing with their eyes, for example, children who are dyslexic, they may be able to process auditory input quicker than processing visual input. They can retain information quickly when they hear it. Have you ever been around a child who is too young to read, yet from their mouth, they blurt fascinating facts? These children are very strong listeners and can store that information easily. Yet, they may have a fantastic visual memory for pictures and describe in detail what is on each page of a story book.

Another example is a child who needs to move their body and enjoys learning through movement and may have exceptional auditory memory. Moving, as reviewed in Chapter 5, can help our auditory system process information better.

These are just examples of how understanding the child's sensory preferences and creating opportunities that match their choices may allow you to teach to a child's strengths rather than their weaknesses. To focus on their weakness would be like giving a child who struggles with dyslexia only a textbook to read and then testing them on that information. They may get through the info, but it would have been a struggle compared to someone who is a proficient reader. Likewise, when lecturing to a student who has difficulty with auditory processing and then questioning their understanding at the end of the lecture, they may have missed parts of the teaching that may have been filled in had they had some visual cues to focus on. The information you teach a child needs to match their abilities and understanding.[16]

> *What is your preferred way to receive information?*
> *How does this relate to your sensory preferences?*

Children also learn by seeing how others interact with the world around them. Children will learn how to treat others by watching their parents, friends, family, or people on television. The way people physically approach others, how they show affection, and how they discipline can all impact how a child learns to treat others.

A child will also learn their vocabulary and how to talk to others by listening to those around them. Language is not innate to us: meaning, it is not something we are born with. We have to learn a language. So, any form of language a child learns, they were exposed to at some point in their life. They can also learn language about themselves as they listen to others speak about them: she is smart, he is silly, they are nightmares, she is dumb. These words can stick with a child as they learn to describe themselves.

I am sure you have all heard stories about a child who seems too young to talk, and right after a parent drops something on the floor and says a swear word, the child repeats it like a parrot. The parent laughs as they are caught off guard, and the child repeats it. The child who mimics your swear word has no idea what the swear word means, nor do they know what they did. Instead, a child will only understand your reaction to whatever they did. If you laugh and smile, they will assume it is something pleasing to you. If you were to be upset or stern, they would feel that it was something you didn't like.

> *Think about what happens when you smile at someone.*
> *Or what happens when you reach out your hand to someone.*

Children start to learn from the reactions of people around them what behaviors will get them attention. Attention shown to a child makes them feel that they belong and have significance in the environment that they are in. Children can get frustrated when they are trying to get an adult's attention and the adult is ignoring them. A small child may be pulling on your leg, or an older child could be whining, but you haven't acknowledged them. Then you drop something and swear like in the last example, and the child swears. If you react by picking them up and giving them attention, you have now made them understand actions that cause a reaction they were looking for.

Children take the information they see, hear, feel, and store into memory banks that tell them how to act when they are around others. Sometimes the memories can be skewed or altered, and their ability to filter information in their brain may not be developed yet. This information forms the ideas that teach children how to treat their teachers, friends, and family.

My son was in daycare when he was little. He had not been around many children before this, as he was an only child at the time. When we put him in daycare, we were shocked, as any new parent would be, that he was bitten by another child in the group. Knowing that the other child was acting out their own sensory needs, we didn't make a big deal about it. What was interesting was that it happened three more times. By the third time it happened, my son started biting other children in the group. With a one-year-old, it is hard to explain to them that biting is wrong, but what was more fascinating was how he picked up this behavior by seeing and experiencing it from others.

Children learn at different rates, and they pick up information around them in a variety of ways. It is hard to unlock the mystery of each of our brain's development, but the more we curiously watch how each child interacts with the world, we can gain an understanding of how to support them.

As a parent, I learn this daily with my children. If I tell my four children to go clean their room, I get four different responses. One child needs me to show them exactly what I mean. Another needs me just to state specifically what it is I need them to do in detail, and then he will do it. Another needs me to write down a list so that she can follow it step by step; otherwise, she doesn't remember what she is supposed to do. The last one follows what everyone else is doing. It is not easy to always accommodate for the child's learning needs, but if I had just said clean your room, one out of four would have completed the task. The same would be true if we didn't accommodate for learning needs within the classroom.

How do you prefer to receive instructions to complete a task?

Should we always focus on children's strengths and never work on their weaker areas? In my opinion, no, but you should use a child's strengths to work on their challenges.

Think about learning a new language. If I gave you a sheet of vocabulary words in that language, but didn't give you a context, it would be hard to remember those words. If I told you all the words were fruits, it might be easier to categorize them in your head. If I showed you a picture of what fruit it was, it would be even easier to match the word to the image and store it in your brain. It comes down to matching our abilities and previous knowledge to help us gain understanding.[16]

Understanding

From the example of my children cleaning their rooms, the first child had difficulty understanding what was being asked of them. What does a "clean room" mean? To one child, if they can see and know where everything is, this could be a clean room, even though it may seem like a disaster to another person. To another child, everything in the room has to have its specific spot, and it needs to be organized by color and size. The term clean is relative to what we understand.

This can be most notable when a child struggles with abstract concepts. If I said to a child, "Be kind," what does that mean? Or if you say to a child, "Just behave," what does that mean?

Have you ever really stopped to think about the language you are using?

Think for a moment about the following words and how they may be perceived as unclear. What do these words mean?

Try harder
Relax
Get along
Be nice
Social distance

The part of our brain that processes abstract concepts can develop at different rates for children and is not fully developed in neurotypical humans till in their 20s. This part of our brain also controls our social skills, impulsivity, planning, and judgments. This is why children often don't understand sarcasm, humor, or idioms. The opposite of abstract is concrete language. Concrete language is the language that is more direct and less likely to get misinterpreted.[12]

Asking a child to get dressed is an abstract term. It doesn't specifically say what you want a child to do and leaves a lot of room for misinterpretation. For instance, a child in their pajamas is technically dressed already because they are wearing clothes. If you wanted a child to get dressed for school, it still might not mean anything different, especially if in the past, they have worn their pajamas to school. To change this to a more concrete term, you need to be specific: "Please get underwear on, a pair of jeans, a t-shirt, a sweater, and some socks." Do you see the difference?

What language do you use that could be misinterpreted?

A lot of learning comes from our understanding of the language and the way we process the language. Saying instructions to children like your shoes are on the wrong feet or that shoe is on the right foot, even if it is the left, can be confusing for many children. The words you use will make a difference.

It can be even more complicated if the language you speak to a child is their second language because information can be lost in translation. For example, you could have a whole conversation about football, only to realize you were talking about American football and they were talking about soccer, also known as football in Europe.

This may look a bit different in a classroom if a teacher in a class asks the students to write a story about their favorite memory. One child may write a three-sentence story, and another may write two pages. They both wrote about their favorite memory, but one child's understanding of the instructions was different from the others understanding of the instructions. If the first child struggles with vocabulary, it may be challenging to find the describing words to elaborate on the story. They may find that the three sentences are enough to trigger an image in their head that brings them back to their favorite time. The child may not be as detail oriented. They feel that they did what the teacher asked them to, which was write a story about their favorite memory. Another child may understand that the teacher wants them to write a story like an essay with an introduction, three paragraphs, and a conclusion. This child may have a very strong vocabulary and may be able to describe to you in detail about their favorite memory. The teacher may look at the second child as following instructions and doing what they were asked and the first child as lazy or uninterested. Now understanding what you learned about abstract and concrete language, what were they asked to do?

Write a story.

What does that mean to you?

It is again about perspective and understanding how a child may experience and interpret the information given to them.

Attaching Knowledge to Meaning

Have you ever tried to build a puzzle without seeing the front of the box?

Have you ever tried to make a recipe without seeing a picture or knowing what you were making?

In their book *Learning How to Learn*, Oakley et al.[17] teach us that we learn better when we can connect information in our brains to understand the concepts and make a path for learning.

Seeing the front of a puzzle box gives us clues about what we are going to put together. When we see a picture of muffins above the directions, it helps us understand our end goal for the recipe.

The same holds true when we are engaging kids in learning. If a child can have a sense of what the lessons are about that we are teaching them, they are more likely to follow along when discussing the details. This can be difficult, as each child may be at a different level of learning or understanding. For example, if you are teaching a child about tennis, showing a video or going out to the court will help a child understand the general idea of tennis.

By providing these previews of learning, we create little hooks in a child's brain. It is almost like we have planted the idea seed so that as we give them more details about the information, it will start to grow in understanding. This can work in many situations and requires that you start with an overview of what you are learning, just like watching the preview of a movie you are about to watch.[17]

Sometimes, we don't have any way to explain a topic, and it can prove more challenging for a child to learn the information. For instance, spelling in the English language has some interesting rules that don't make sense. For example, a mouse in the plural is mice, and a goose is geese, but a moose is just moose. It is hard sometimes for our brain to grasp information if we don't have a little bit of an anchor to hook it on to, to stick the information in the right spot so that we can retrieve it again.

This is when it is imperative to understand the children you are working with. To associate learning with something that they already recognize or understand means that you need to know what they are familiar with. There are analogies that we use to help students learn how to print their letters. One compares letters to a house. A tall letter goes to the second floor, a hanging letter goes to the basement, and all the rest stay on the main floor. If children live in an apartment and have never been in a house, will they understand what this means?

Likewise, if you use an analogy or compare a cell in biology to how a car operates, this would be wonderful for someone who loves cars and understands the car's parts. Yet for someone like me, a car is a box with four wheels that gets me from A to B.

Working at the child's understanding and level of knowledge is essential. Every child will develop at different rates and have different amounts of knowledge planted in their brains. If you can find the hooks that they already have, you can start to build pathways to those hooks that will get stronger and stronger all the time. If they don't have the hooks yet, that is where you need to start. Begin with something they understand and then build onto it. Just like building a house, the foundation is the most important part.[17]

Mindset

Remember the conversation we had previously about fixed and growth mindsets in adults? The same applies to understanding how children learn. If children believe that they will never understand math, they are stuck in a fixed mindset. It is the limiting belief in their capabilities. Every test they get back that they do poorly on will be a reminder that they are bad at math. It is challenging to get a child out of a fixed mindset, yet it is vital for their growth and learning potential.

In her book *Mindset*, Carol Dweck[7] said that children are often sorted based on their grades and past achievements in schools, but this is built off of a fixed mindset. The things we have done in the past only tell us about what we have achieved so far; it doesn't tell us what we are capable of.[7]

The opposite of the fixed mindset is a growth mindset: the belief that we can continually learn and grow. With a growth mindset, you can create opportunities to learn in all different areas with the right support and the right conditions.[7]

Mindset plays a crucial role in understanding how children learn, and it is not only their belief in themselves but also those around them believing in them. By creating opportunities for them to learn, they can continue to reach their potential.

If you have a child stuck in a fixed mindset, spend time working on developing the growth mindset. You can do this by changing the language you use with the child, increasing their understanding of how the brain develops, or challenging them to learn new things.

Motivation

Motivation also affects a child's ability to learn. What if I told you that you could be the next person to go to the moon if you could write a paper on the solar system?

Would you do it?

Maybe, but maybe not. It will depend if you are interested in going to the moon, and if it's not important to you, it may not motivate you to try hard or even write the paper at all.

If you are a car person and I told you that you could win your favorite car if you could write a paper about all its details, chances are you would write the essay. A child who understands cars will be able to provide a great deal of detailed information. They will be able to expand on that information, especially if they have some motivation.

Motivation is often attached to our personal desires. We are each motivated by different things. Something that will motivate me will be different from something that motivates you. My daughter loves gum and will do anything to get her hands on some. I don't like gum. Reflecting on Chapter 5, it is probably due to the auditory sensitivity I have to chewing, so it is not something that motivates me. When my daughter needs to get something done, she will do it to get a piece of gum. She is only six years old, so in her world, that is a big deal. Will my older children be motivated by gum like my six-year-old? Most likely not.

External motivators are objects or people that we attach value or importance to and that encourage us to accomplish a goal. Our world is built around numerous external motivators for adults. They are always striving for a better job, a bigger house, or a new car. I often see children do an activity to gain a new toy or a fun treat, but more often, I notice their motivation to be seen, loved, accepted, or out of fear of losing one of those connections.

I recently watched the movie *Wonder*[18] with my children. This movie, although fictitious, describes events that many children encounter. The main character in the film, Auggie, was born with a craniofacial disorder known as Treacher Collins syndrome. This syndrome alters the development of facial features and often requires many surgeries. Auggie begins school, and as the movie viewer, you get a first-hand account of what he sees when people look at him. You see people's facial reactions, students moving out of his way snickering, and you see parents pull their kids closer to them. He encounters many different experiences, including overcoming people's assumptions that because he looks different, it means he can't learn or understand. You watch as other children in his class are pressured by their friends to make fun of him so that they can be a part of the "cool kids" group, or a child is left out and made fun of because she became friends with Auggie.[18]

This doesn't just happen in the movies. This depiction was bringing to light the truth about children's motivations. The way we treat others can be motivated by internal and external factors, such as wanting to feel accepted or belonging to a group of friends. It happens in all our schools, on playgrounds, in families, and in groups.

If we are not somehow motivated by our learning, it is harder for us to have the energy, effort, or focus on staying engaged. When working with a child, we can't choose their motivation for them. Each child will have something different that motivates them to do an activity.

Think of a kindergarten classroom that gets stickers for behavior. Each child gets a sticker when they have had a good day at school. A few children may be motivated by this, but most children who would get stickers for good behavior would have acted that way without the sticker reward, and the children who never get a sticker are most likely not motivated by the sticker's reward, so it doesn't impact them at all. This is where spending the time to understand a child and their motivations will affect how and why they behave the way they do.[19]

Have you ever heard a child did poorly at math, but grew up to be fantastic at managing money? A job, money, lifestyle can all be motivators for people.

Consider someone who struggled with spelling, sequencing, organizing, but was exceptional at saving lives as a paramedic? Desiring a life of impact, high stress, and excitement can also be motivators.

What is a motivator for you to get your work done?

When you can connect yourself to something that motivates you, it is easier to accomplish that goal. External goals, depending on how big they are, can also lead to disappointments. Think about a child who always dreamed about being a professional hockey player. Each year they work harder and harder and pour all of their efforts and energies into reaching their goal. What happens if they never become a professional hockey player? What will they think about all the years they worked hard, gained more skills, and achieved success? They may feel it was all lost in the disappointment of not reaching their goal.

The same can be said for a child who worked hard in school and played violin in the orchestra only to gain their parent's love and attention. They focused only on pleasing others as their motivation, rather than doing what they were passionate about or what motivated them. In the end, the effort they put into pleasing others may not give them the fulfillment they desired.

Yet motivation doesn't even need to be external; there can be internal motivators. Internal motivators are when you are motivated by a desire to gain knowledge or to be a better person. There is extensive psychology behind internal and external motivators.

Teaching children how to be motivated by internal motivators, such as the goal to learn something new or become proficient at a skill and celebrate this success, is key in helping kids become confident adults.

> *What do you do to please others?*
> *What would you do if you only need to do it for yourself?*

Internal motivators are goals we set for ourselves that involve our ability to grow continually. It is not based on what others think or how it will change others' opinions; it is about how it will make us better. Trying to help children learn and build this skill will connect them with who they authentically are and their own hopes and dreams.

The Education System and Learning

Take a moment to think about your elementary school. Try to picture one of your classrooms. What did it look like? Did you have desks? Was your room full of other children? Did your teacher have pictures and images on the walls, and did they use a chalkboard?

Chances are, we all have a similar recollection of our schools. A classroom was full of desks with hard plastic chairs. A blackboard at the front of the classroom. Bells that rang for lunch and recess and lots of kids moving about in the hallways.

The interesting fact is that schools haven't changed much over the last 50 years. The introduction of technology has changed chalkboards into whiteboards or smart boards, but the physical environment is the same. The challenge is that we have learned so much about how children learn, yet our education system often doesn't match students' needs.

By creating the conversation about each child's unique story, we will understand how we can create an environment for learning that matches a child's sensory and learning needs and ensure that each caregiver or teacher involved with a child takes the time to connect with the child they are working with. My hope is that as we collectively learn to recognize this information, we will make decisions about the future that will work towards creating environments that match their needs.

Connecting to the Child

How do you connect with a child to motivate them?

How can you incorporate how a child learns into their story?

It all starts with building a bond with the child so they know that they belong and are significant.

Start with believing in a growth mindset of acknowledging that all children can learn. They may not learn at the same rate, but they all have the ability to learn new information and skills.[7] Then recognizing and understanding how a child experiences the world around them through their sensory system will give us clues into how they process information. Once you can understand this, you can focus on the child's strengths and build off the knowledge they already have to help them learn. Create a space that accepts people for who they are and acknowledges their learning differences.

What if a child doesn't feel like they belong or struggles with sensory overload? What if a child acts out, throws fits, or runs away? How does their behavior become part of their story? In the next chapter, I will look at what causes behaviors and how, sometimes, behaviors are mistaken goals or unsolved problems that are the outward display of internal struggles.

Chapter Reflections

1. What are the different learning strengths?
2. What is the difference between concrete and abstract language?
3. Why is it important to understand how a child interprets language?
4. Why is it valuable to attach new learning to information we already know?
5. What is the difference between internal and external motivators?

7 Understanding Behaviors

Often people will fabricate a story in their mind about a child by the way that they act. A child throwing himself on the ground in a grocery store or a child crying during a haircut may make people think this child has no discipline or needs to "grow up." At this point in the book, you should understand how much more there is to a child and how complex each child is. The story of who they are is more than just their name.

A child is a product of who the caregivers are, their biology, and the environment they are growing up in. A child's sense of belonging and love can impact their connection to themselves and others. How they experience the world through their sensory system and how they learn will affect how their bodies and minds engage daily. There is so much information that a child needs to process to be a part of the world that it is not surprising when they sometimes feel overwhelmed. I am sure each person reading this can understand that feeling. The days when your sensory system is heightened, sounds bother you, lights feel too bright, it feels like no one understands you, and you are tasked with an assignment that you don't know where to begin.

When a child acts out or shows a sense of frustration, sometimes it can be seen as purposeful and intentional by those around them. Yet their behaviors can be a child's way of communicating their frustrations and emotions. Language development and emotional intelligence can occur at different rates, and therefore, children can react without fully understanding the impact of their reactions. The part of our brain that controls the body's response and rational processing of our environment often doesn't fully develop until we are in our 20s, and for some, it may not fully develop.[12] Therefore, behaviors can also be a body's way of dealing with stress that a child can't yet fully identify. How adults around the child react when they are misbehaving can escalate the behaviors, encourage it, or help them learn to regulate the behavior's cause.

What Are Behaviors?

We often describe behaviors as the outward response to internal feelings. Behaviors can be positive or negative. When we have hit our first baseball or

DOI: 10.4324/9781003166405-7

learned to ride our bike, we see the joy and excitement that we display as positive behaviors. We could be jumping up and down, screaming with pleasure, or smiling from ear to ear.

Listening in class, doing our homework, helping out at home, or doing the task we are asked to do are also seen as positive behaviors because they are in line with what is expected of us.

When things don't go our way, and we are frustrated, angry, or upset, we tend to misbehave. This display of negative behaviors can range through many actions, such as withdrawing, fighting, restlessness, rebelling, inattentive, or resisting.

Why are we encouraged to show behaviors that express only happy, joyful moments and often discouraged to exhibit behaviors associated with being frustrated, angry, or upset?

In his book *Self-Reg,* Dr. Stuart Shanker[20] refers to these as behavioral signs of a person being depleted of energy with tensions heightened. Being in this state can trigger what he refers to as a stress cycle. The challenge is that we can all have ongoing stress cycles that can interact with someone else who is under stress, making ours amplified.[20]

Jackson did not like school at all. He would come each day, put his head down on his desk, and avoid eye contact. He would grunt when the teacher asked him a question and would rarely participate. On most days, his teacher would be upbeat, encouraging, and creatively try to engage him. On occasion, his teacher would have those days when everything was just a challenge. On those days, she would express her frustration with Jackson's lack of effort and engagement. Not even raising her voice, but her demeanor had changed. It was enough that Jackson could sense it. At this point, Jackson would escalate and push the desk, knock over chairs, and walk out of the classroom.

Jackson's stress was already heightened before school even began. Not from the school, but from other situations going on in his life. He barely had food to eat coming to school, and his family struggled to pay the bills. He lived in a one-bedroom apartment with his three siblings and his mom. He was up late at night, had difficulty sleeping, and was exhausted most days. He had trouble recognizing letters and numbers and had difficulty staying focused. It was a lot for a child in second grade. Any sense of additional tension around him was enough to push Jackson into an angry state.

Every aspect of a person's life can affect the other. Like the CMOP-E[4] I referred to in Chapter 2, we are a being made up of our person (i.e., physical, cognitive, and affective beings), our occupation (i.e., the activities we do), and our environment. Figure 2.1 in Chapter 2 depicts this model. Stress in any of these pieces will have implications on the rest of the aspects.[4] This can even affect our lives as adults.

Have you ever had a struggle with a co-worker at a job?

Work can be a stressful place. If you didn't see eye to eye with your co-worker, it could make going to your job more stressful. When you left work and went home, did it then affect your relationships at home? Did you have difficulty sleeping? Difficulty doing your leisure activities?

Your family members may have felt that you were crabby. They may have tried to help you out of your slump, but what may have happened is that your stress affected everyone else's level of tension. The stress from one person can increase the stress from another.

If the main stressor is not identified, it is hard to help someone regain balance in their life. Often what happens is the focus is on the behaviors that are prominent on a daily basis. Dealing with the behaviors one at a time could include something like you getting sleeping medication to help with sleeping and starting counselling for relationships at home. These approaches did not recognize what caused the stress, just the outcome of the stress.

The same could be true for a child such as Jackson. If his teacher became upset at him each day, demanding eye contact or continuously sending him to the principal's office for not listening, she would have been missing the stressor that was making him behave the way he was.

What we see as outward displays of emotions in one area of life may only be the tip of an iceberg of other things that could potentially be going on.

Where Do Behaviors Come From?

What triggers behaviors is an internal change that creates an outward expression. We are often unconcerned with children who are expressing behaviors of joy and excitement, so the term we should focus on is misbehaviors—behaviors that are viewed as more negative or against what is expected. Often, a misbehavior is an age-appropriate expression of frustration, anger, and upset that we would expect to see in children. They are a child's response to a situation outside of their control, and oftentimes, these responses are because they don't have the skills or language to deal with it. A hungry or tired child can misbehave because they may not recognize their body's way of telling them this information. Often, adults forget that this is a normal reaction from children, and this can cause the anger and frustration in a caregiver's response to the child.[9]

Like Jackson in the last section, his behaviors resulted from unstable home conditions that affected his ability to focus, tolerate, and control his emotions in the classroom. It is important to understand that children would control their behavior if they could. This is something that Dr. Greene emphasizes in his book *Lost at School*.[19] When a child has a task they are expected to participate in or complete and don't have the skills to do what they are supposed to, it creates a gap in their ability to perform. Dr. Greene refers to these as behaviors resulting from lagging skills and unsolved problems. A caregiver expects that a child can perform at a certain level, but when they can't, the frustration often comes from the child not meeting these expectations.[19] It can seem that the child is refusing to do the task, but instead they don't have the skills to do it yet.

Do you ever wish that you could control your anger or frustration?

It is not easy to change our moods, our thoughts, or our actions, even when we feel we have the skills we need. So, believing that children will control their behaviors, if they can, is important because it takes the focus off the child's motives and moves it to their lack of skills or abilities. Remember, our ability to reason, make good decisions, and control impulsivity is the last part of our brain to develop and may not develop till our mid-20s. I repeat this because of our belief that kids have the skills necessary to control their behavior or even understand their actions is coming from adults who have already developed these skills.[12] This is why it is vital to recognize how the information we covered in the last three chapters is important to understand, as it can impact a child's behaviors. The struggles a child experiences can be because of their response to the sensory environment, a disconnect with learning, or their struggle to belong and feel loved.

Sensory Overload

A child who is having difficulties processing all of the sensory information around them may experience a sense of overwhelm or overload. Imagine you had 10 people talking to you all at the same time, while the fire alarm is going off and the dog is barking. This scenario would be overwhelming.

When our brain perceives a stressor or information that it doesn't understand or has an over-response to, like I discussed in Chapter 5 on sensory information, our brain will trigger an instinctive protective reaction. This response activates our primitive brain, which doesn't include reasoning and rationalization. Instead, it may trigger a fight-or-flight response. The fight response is displayed as a power struggle—arguing, defensive, aggressive—and the flight response is often expressed as a withdrawal, running away, hiding, or inability to communicate.[9]

Ahmed was a child in a kindergarten class who would get so overwhelmed by the classroom noises that when it became too much, he would bury his head under pillows, or rock his body, or make loud noises to himself. The teachers found that they were unable to comfort him when he was overwhelmed. This was because Ahmed had gone into his primitive brain and had withdrawn as a form of self-protection. He was using his body movements and humming combined with his withdrawal to allow his brain a chance to calm down.

When the frustration in class turns to anger, the power struggle or fight response will activate. Damien was in Grade 2 and struggled with learning. He was often overwhelmed by what was being asked of him. He was also tactile defensive. When someone would come close to him or touch him, he would explode with rage. On occasion, he would knock over furniture or people. There were instances when classrooms needed to be evacuated for the safety of the other children.

Each child will react in different ways. A child who is sensitive to lights in a classroom or has difficulty with smells of laundry detergent or foods may find school overwhelming daily. A child who has vestibular insecurity and feels as though they are walking on a rocking boat all day may feel overwhelmed whenever they need to move about the classroom, or they may resist going out for recess. The brain can have difficulty processing all that is going. Each of these children's behaviors can be perceived as defiant, yet the underlying reason is far from defiance.

Combining a child's sensory preferences with transitions or changes in schedules and routines can also be stressful for children if they have not yet developed that skill. This can lead to frustration and a lack of ability to control emotions, especially when they are in a space where they are comfortable and calm and not wanting to leave. Think about how hard it is to get out of bed some mornings when your bed is cozy and warm or pivoting a busy day to take care of an ill relative. It can make you feel out of sorts even as adults.

It can also happen with a child who is so engrossed in video games that they can't transition away from the games. The video games may be providing some calming aspects for the child or maybe a world that is easier for the child to control. Video games and technology have been designed to play into our brain's reward system and can be calming to the senses. It is why it is so hard for even adults to moderate their technology use.

Children may also feel overwhelmed when they are overscheduled. When a child is taken from one activity to another, a child may have a limit of what they can tolerate. If a child can't express this limit, they may resist going to activities or have a meltdown when they get to the program.

Understanding how behaviors can come from overwhelming sensory inputs is essential to understand a child's story. If you forget about the sensory concerns, go back to Chapter 5. By recognizing a child's preferences, you can understand what they try to avoid and what they crave, and the information can help to create the best environment for a child to learn to find balance.

Our bodies are only in a state of calm when we can find balance within our sensory system. This is known as self-regulation, which is so important. I will spend the next chapter going into more detail.

Learning Needs

As I reviewed in Chapter 6, the way a child learns can be related to sensory needs, understanding, and motivation. If a child struggles with any of these aspects, learning can be challenging and may result in the body feeling overwhelmed by what is being asked of it.

I remember sitting in a university statistics class. It was a first-year class and mandatory for all students. Math was not my strongest subject, but I could hold my own. However, this professor of statistics made me feel as though he was talking in a foreign language. Each week, I would sit in class and look around at others to see if they could understand what he was saying. I was unable to process what he was saying. I remember distinctly getting that uneasy feeling of not wanting to be in that class anymore, wanting to get up and walk out. It would get to the point that my mind was focused only on planning my escape route.

Was there a class or a time where you struggled with learning a new skill?

When there is a disconnect in a child's ability to learn, they cannot stay focused or attend to any of the information. They become disengaged and may even be planning their escape, just like I was. The child may be lacking the skills needed to participate in the lesson. On good days when the rest of their world is functioning in a neutral state, they may be able to stay in class and control their desire to escape. Yet, if they come to school, as Dr. Shanker referred to as depleted of energy, their ability to handle any high-stress situation may cause them to go into a stress response or misbehavior.[20]

Acknowledging a child's ability to learn and understand information, combined with their motivation to learn, will impact how they respond in learning situations. A child may function well at school in gym class or recess, but may struggle when they are pushed out of their comfort zone and required to do more than the child feels capable of doing.

Abe was in Grade 2 and loved to learn new information, but struggled with any written work. His vocabulary was very strong, and his printing was legible, but the speed he could write did not match the rate at which his brain was processing information. Abe could tell you a great story with lots of details, but he would get frustrated writing one sentence on paper. His teacher would comment on his lack of effort and grade him poorly. This sense of frustration would bottle up inside, and he would spend his afternoons irritable and angry. Abe didn't have the skill to get his story on paper, but he didn't know how to explain that to his teacher.

If we remember that a child would do well if they could, it changes the perspective on children who struggle with learning. What resources and support can we give them that will meet them where they are at? What can we do to create an environment that encourages and promotes a love for learning?

Sense of Belonging and Love

In combination with a child's ability to process the sensory world and engage in learning, a child innately desires to feel that they belong or are loved and are capable, as I discussed in Chapter 4. If this connection is not felt, children can behave in ways that they mistakenly believe will give them this attention. According to Rudolf Dreikurs, there are four mistaken ways a child believes that they belong. These four beliefs focus on attention, power, revenge, and inadequacy. For this book's purpose, I will only cover the notion that these beliefs exist, are the basis for some behaviors, and can create a disconnect for a child within many situations.[21]

If a child believes they need to fight for attention because then they will belong, they may seek any attention from a caregiver or friend, whether good or bad. Think about an older sibling who just had a new baby brother. The older sibling received all the attention from their parents before the new baby's arrival. The sibling then watched in wonder as the parents now turned all their attention onto the baby. Every time the baby cries, the parents jump up. They spend time rocking the baby to sleep and changing his diaper whenever it is soiled. Whenever the sibling's parents come to play with him, if his baby sibling cries, the attention gets diverted. The older sibling begins to recognize what behaviors get the most attention. Think about what happens when an adult is focused on their phone. A child will often fight for a parent's attention by misbehaving.[21]

> *Think back to when you were young. Was there a child in your life who captured all the attention because of unpleasurable behavior? A sibling? A child in a class? Camp?*

Unpleasant behavior captures attention all the time. Look at the news, read the paper. The focus is often on what is going wrong in the world rather than what is going right. What are we teaching children about who gets the attention?

Children can also, according to Dreikurs,[21] struggle with control and power. Think about a situation you were in as a child or adult where you were told what to do and never given a chance to share your opinion or view. Did you feel that you were valued in this situation? Did you feel that your opinion mattered? It reminds me of the military setting and how the hierarchy of the ranking officials determines how you must behave. Your opinion and input don't matter as long as you do as you are told.[21]

A child may struggle with being told what to do or when they don't get their way because they feel belonging is tied to who has power and control. This mistaken belief can come from the fear of losing control or of not wanting to be controlled. If someone has ever hurt us in the past, we can build up a subconscious guard that we won't let anyone control us. We protect ourselves by continually seeking to take away any power over us.

Ramona was in Grade 9. She was living with her mom; her parents had divorced due to some history of physical abuse. Ramona did not like to be bound by rules. She did her own thing every day at school. The school Ramona went to was uniformed, and although she wore the uniform, she would add a flare that was against the dress code. Her constant power struggle with authority was draining on the teachers and principal at the school. Ramona was not going to be told what to do, and the stronger the punishment, the more she got her back up. Ramona's history played a lot into her inability to let her guard down. She had watched her dad come home in fits of rage and take his anger out on her mom. For years, she watched the vulnerability and power struggle ensued in that relationship. It impacted how she would let others treat her. She would not let her guard down.

The stronger resistance was displayed by Ramona, the worse the power struggle. She was unable to recognize why she was so resistant to authority because it was so ingrained in her subconscious that she did not even understand where it came from. She didn't know what it meant to be in a mutually respectful relationship. She only knew what she had experienced in her own upbringing. This power struggle made Ramona feel that she didn't belong. If she couldn't have some control, she felt that she had no significance.

If a child was ever made to feel that they were not good enough to belong, they might feel the need to retaliate against or have revenge on those who fit in or belong.[21] Jamie was in Grade 8; he was behind in school and had difficulty staying on task or following what the teacher asked. He felt the teacher didn't like him being in class, and he didn't want his classmates to think he was "stupid." Instead, he chose to pick on other kids in class. Jamie would be disruptive in class and would say sarcastic remarks to the teacher while the teacher was trying to give the class instructions. Jamie would try to make it hard for the teacher because Jamie believed the teacher didn't want him there anyway.

Jamie's situation was complicated, just like Ramona's. Ramona's belief stemmed from her experiences of her upbringing and how she treated those around her. Jamie's learning needs affected his comfort level in class. Despite the teacher's efforts to help Jamie, Jamie assumed the teacher's focus on helping was because she was disappointed. It impacted how the teacher and other kids in the class were treated. If Jamie didn't belong in the class, others shouldn't belong either.

The last belief by Dreikurs was that the child feels that they are not worthy of belonging. I, unfortunately, have met children in my career who have been told by their caregivers that they are useless and incompetent. These children have lost the desire to try because, to them, it won't make a difference anyway. They are disengaged from activities and unmotivated. Their withdrawal behavior won't go away without first creating a belief in their self-worth and belonging.[21]

Curtis, in Grade 3, couldn't tie his shoes yet. His teacher didn't think he could learn anything, as Curtis was so disengaged from classwork, he hardly turned anything in. Curtis did not come from a very supportive home environment; his parents were busy with work and other responsibilities and had little time for him. Curtis had significant learning challenges as well as decreased eye–hand coordination, which made any activities with paper and pencil difficult as well as activities like tying his shoes. Using strategies to help him in therapy sessions, he was able to tie his own shoes successfully. His teacher's lack of excitement when he returned to class brought back the bitter disappointment that he felt daily and emphasized that he shouldn't bother trying because no one cared.

The mistaken beliefs about how to achieve belonging give us an idea of how the brain connection can influence our outward behaviors. Once you understand the belief behind a child's behavior, you can support them in creating new ideas of socially useful ways of belonging. Dreikurs would often express that a child who is misbehaving is a child who is discouraged.[21]

The way we feel loved can also impact our sense of belonging. The love languages that we covered in Chapter 4 show us how unique a child's interpretation of love is and how sensitive a child could be if they are not shown love from any caregivers. In the same realm, if you understand a child's love language, then you can create a connection that makes a child feel that they belong.[11]

Understanding the child's whole story and putting together the pieces will help you understand why certain behaviors exist and also how to help the child work through these mistaken beliefs about themselves and others. If the child was disciplined for the outward display of behavior that was expressed without understanding the stressors or cause, then the focus would have not helped to resolve the mistaken beliefs.

The Way a Child Expresses Behaviors

So far in this chapter, I have discussed the motive behind the action. How a child physically displays behaviors can be learned behavior and can be a lack of control. Just like children pick up language from their parents, the way parents react in happy situations and stressful situations will be what a child will store in their memory. Likewise, what they see in movies and television, as well as from other classmates, will influence some of their behaviors. Behavior is often learned through what we experience and what we see. Suppose a child comes from a household that has a lot of yelling in the home. A child might learn that you may need to raise your voice or make loud noises to get your way. Likewise, parents who swear a lot or talk degradingly to each other may impact how a child speaks to and treats others.

Just like my son who was exposed to biting in daycare, the child in his daycare used biting to get his toy. My son mimicked the behavior when he was at home, as he thought it would help him get his way.

Children need to see healthy examples from their caregivers about how to interact with others. When children don't learn how to relate well to others, they may try to control others, engaging in such things as bullying.[11]

Sometimes children internalize the way that they feel, and instead of having outward displays, their stress may manifest into internal symptoms. Even from experience with children I have worked with, I have seen many children who experience stomach pains, headaches, joint pains, and anxiety when they are feeling overwhelmed or tasked with an activity that they don't have the skills for. When these symptoms exist, it is always important to rule out a physical cause, but it is also valuable to be curious about other factors that may be causing these symptoms.

Why Do We Look at Some Behaviors so Negatively?

We look at behaviors with a negative lens often when it affects us personally or fear that the behavior reflects our abilities as parents, caregivers, teachers, or therapists.

Sometimes, our personal response to behaviors is because they hit close to home, which means that our sensory preferences can also affect our reactions. I am sensitive to sound, so a screaming child is more challenging for me to tolerate. Especially when I need to focus on something, I cannot handle even the slightest noise, or I lose complete focus. Sounds are a trigger for me. For others, touch may be a trigger. If you are upset and someone touches you, it may be too much for your sensory system to handle at that moment. Our own sensory experiences as well as our past experiences can trigger a negative reaction to some behaviors.

Our expectations for how a child should behave, look, and act create an often-unreachable goal. As a parent, we hope that our children will be the perfect version of ourselves. They will not struggle the way we did, and they will know how to interact appropriately with others. When this doesn't happen, we judge any misbehavior negatively. Our disappointments are a result of unmet expectations that were often unrealistic. The same can be said for a therapist or caregiver with unrealistic therapeutic goals or a teacher with unreachable learning objectives. Our focus may be on our expectations and not those of the child.

Comparison is also a moderator for how we judge behaviors.

Have you ever looked at social media and compared your life to others? Have you thought about how perfect someone's life seems or how well-behaved their children are?

Their house is immaculate, their skin smooth, and their children are happy. When we compare ourselves or our children to others, we lose sight of what makes them who they are. We live in a world, now more than ever, that has set high expectations and ideals that are unreachable. We strive towards often-staged photos, and the world is trending towards outwards expressions of approval rather than internal satisfaction. When we have these expectations in our mind, anything less than ideal can make us feel less competent or disappointed.

Fear can also play a factor in our reaction to our children's behaviors. I worked with a mother who was so fearful that her child would get hurt when they tried to walk that she would continuously sit her child down if they tried to stand up. The child stopped trying to stand over time and would cry and flail if someone encouraged him to walk. He, therefore, had difficulty progressing to walking. Was this child incapable of walking, or was it the fear of the parent that held them back? The behavior that this child displayed was a result of the parent's fear.

Where that fear came from and what transcended this situation is vital to understand.

As a child, I lost my front tooth when I was around nine months old. I knocked it on a coffee table, and it fell out. My mother took the tooth, rushed me to the dentist, and tried to get the dentist to place the tooth back in. The dentist said he couldn't do it. For the next seven years, I had one front tooth missing in all my photos. I recall being made fun of when I was little and self-conscious of it. When I had my own children, my third child knocked his tooth out on the night table next to my bed. He was 11 months old. All I could think is that I didn't want him to go through what I went through. I grabbed the tooth off the ground, which thankfully was clean, laid him on the bed, and put the tooth back in the gaping hole in his mouth. My behavior at that moment had a direct correlation to what happened when I was little.

The mother who didn't want her child to fall while learning to walk had some belief that she needed to protect them. Maybe it was a similar tooth story, or perhaps somewhere along the line, a child she knew or heard of had injured themselves. The memories and the experience that we have create a response in us and affect our behaviors towards the children we work with. This can then affect their behaviors.

Not only can we have fear of a child getting hurt, but we can also fear that a child will hurt someone or themselves—a fear that a child will not be success-ful or that they will be lazy or not be independent. Parents may fear that their child may make them look bad as parents. A parent may blame themselves for a child's behaviors and may internalize the feelings of self-doubt, shame, guilt, and anger, which spirals the situation and doesn't allow them to see that the negative behaviors from children are not a reflection of them. The parent may be missing the stressor that is affecting their child.

Even teachers, doctors, entrepreneurs, and leaders in organizations can fear someone thinking they are not capable. When fear comes into play, we are more sensitive to any behaviors that may make us feel like the story we told ourselves, such as that we are incompetent, is true.[9] For example, if a coworker questions something that you have done, it may trigger your fear that they think you are not capable or in control and immediately make you defensive.

> *Have you ever told yourself a story that you weren't good at something, and a comment from someone reiterates that for you?*

I had a client recently who witnessed her son in a classroom with his teacher. The teacher had given the class instructions to sit down, put up their hand, and she would call on each of them to come to the front and hand in their agenda. Her son only heard the words come to the front and hand in your agenda, and so that is what he did. Because he didn't follow directions, she got upset at him. The teacher assumed he was disrespectful, so she tried to get him to return to his seat and try it again, but instead, the child got angry and ran out of the class-room. The teacher was fearful that if she let him get away with not following the instructions this time, she would lose control of the class. Her fear skewed her ability to see the child's inability to recall more than two-step instructions. Her instinctive reaction made her look at the child's behavior more negatively than may have been necessary.

Some of this fear can come from past negative experiences that we have had in our own story. We may not want a child to experience something that we endured, whether it be the result of abuse or trauma. What if you were criticized by your parents for the way you look? Your parents commented on your weight, your appearance, your clothes. You became so self-conscious about yourself that you developed a low self-esteem growing up. You are so acutely aware of how others look at you that you make choices and subconsciously react to others due to your own low self-esteem. It results in you controlling anything that you can control. If we have children or work with children, we again can set those unrealistic expectations. Then when a child refuses to follow your rules and misbehaves, it may cause your reaction to be inappropriate for the action. The control we instill on a child will affect how they react to others and will impact how they react if they become parents themselves.

Our past experiences affect our tolerance for behaviors, but our current mental capacity can also come into play. If someone is struggling with depression or anxiety, tolerance for behavior can be affected. Emotions are heightened, and the focus is only on survival. The ability to balance outwardly what is going on is limited, and therefore, we need to create boundaries, seek help, and acknowledge the effect of our own capacity for judgment of the behavior.

The reaction to some behaviors comes down again to perspective. How each person responds and reacts will be different, and that is why some people can tolerate some behaviors better than others.

How to Be Proactive When Looking at Behaviors

To be proactive means to recognize the potential for something to happen and be prepared in advance. In regard to behaviors, this means understanding the belief I covered earlier in this chapter that a child will do well if they can, and then believe that a child is capable if given the right tools and skills. This follows the growth mindset that a child can and will be able to learn new skills.[19]

Try to understand the underlying causes of the behavior, whether it be sensory, learning, or a desire for belonging and being considered significant. Then work to set up the environment to meet the child's needs. This environment should make the child feel safe, that they belong and are significant. This will be covered in Chapter 9. A child also needs to have the support, the skills, and resources to know how to deal with situations that come up. For older children, including them in the solution is an essential part of gaining their cooperation. In the *Explosive Child* by Dr. Ross Greene,[22] he refers to the solution to the situation as Plan B. It is not what you would instinctively do as a caregiver, which is often based on the fear and control response, which he calls Plan A. Instead, Plan B focuses on what the child's trying to tell you through their behavior. Then the child is included in the plan. If you work with the child, you will understand their perspective, and they will feel a greater sense of belonging.[22]

Never limit someone by their diagnosis, their behavior, or your personal beliefs. Recognize that these beliefs may come from a place of protection, but having a proactive approach means believing in a child's potential. When you believe in someone's potential, you can make them feel like they are capable of so much more. It is in this belief that children excel and soar.

If we believe that a child can walk, we need to let them get up and try. Even though they may fall, it is through this experience that they will eventually learn. We don't let them learn to walk over sharp rocks and near the edge of a cliff. Instead, we set them in an environment where they will not endanger themselves even if they fall. Through this safe environment, a child will learn the skills and eventually be able to confidently walk to the point that they can handle the rougher terrain.

A child learning to walk needs encouragement and sometimes a little support to get back up, but like the mom who continuously sat her child back down, if we don't believe a child will be successful, they won't believe in themselves.

Acknowledge that it is okay to have feelings. It is okay to be upset, sad, angry, or frustrated. These emotions create energy in us to often promote development and change. A baby who is learning to crawl often does so because they are so frustrated that they can't reach their toy that they reach just a little bit further and eventually move. A basketball player who misses the basket will practice just a little more to improve their accuracy. Feelings also help indicate that our body is overwhelmed, and we may need to find a way to regulate our emotions. Learning how our body is speaking to us can help us understand how to self-regulate. It is important for a child to navigate an ever-changing world. In the next chapter, I will go into detail about what self-regulation means, why it is important, and how to help children develop these skills. Self-regulation becomes one of the keys to helping a child manage their stress and the environmental influences from their sensory and learning needs.

Our goal is not to change a child to fit society; our goal is to understand a child to create a world where they belong.

Chapter Reflections

1. What are behaviors?
2. What is the benefit of looking at children through the lens that they would "behave if they could"?
3. How can learning differences turn into behaviors?
4. As adults, why are we more sensitive to some behaviors?
5. How can we be proactive when looking at behaviors?

8 Helping a Child Find Balance

Once you have gathered enough information to understand a child's story as it relates to how they experience and react to the world, the next step is to teach them how to find a sense of balance or a place of calm. A child sitting in class feeling overwhelmed by what they are trying to learn might explode in anger, or a child who wasn't allowed a snack before dinner may cry in overwhelm because of the hunger their body is identifying, or a child who lies in bed all day may struggle with energy and initiation. We want to identify the behavior and have strategies to help before we get to the point where the brain can't function very well anymore and our primitive brain kicks in, which either puts up a fight or withdraws.

If we understand how we get to that point where we feel overwhelmed, we can then understand what is referred to as our "triggers." As adults, we often don't think about what we do in these situations anymore. If we are feeling stressed, we often change our environment to help us feel more in control. Although we may not remember how we learned what helped us find our preferred balance state, we tend to do the same few activities to reach that balance.

Whenever I run a group for parents, I want them first to understand how they experience the world and what they do to help themselves. It can give clarity to what we are asking our children to do. One question that I ask is:

When you are feeling overwhelmed, what helps you get into a calm state?

What is always amazing to me is the array of answers I may get in any given group. Here is a list of a few of the responses:

Scroll on their phone
Go for a run
Have a cup of tea
Take a bath
Call a friend
Watch television
Take a nap
Read a book

DOI: 10.4324/9781003166405-8

Bake
Work in my garden
Take a break

Each person had a different activity that would restore that sense of balance for them, and many said that the other suggestions would not help them. When we changed the question to "How do you get settled to go to sleep?", they again had a wide array of answers and habitual practices each night.

My next question to the group was: "How did you learn that these activities would help you find calm?" Many couldn't remember when they started, but they knew that they enjoyed the feeling these activities brought. What the parents learned by doing this activity was that they often subconsciously regulate their feelings, and they no longer have to think about it. Children are just learning what works for them, which can be challenging to figure out, and they often need support to help guide them through learning how to self-regulate.

Charlene hated wearing her socks. She could not find a comfortable pair. Her mom would not let her go to school until she had her socks on. Every morning, Charlene would resist getting ready for school and would make the family late, as she would throw herself on the floor and cry that she wasn't going to school. It wasn't just the socks; there were only a few pairs of pants that Charlene would wear and only one type of t-shirt. Getting dressed was stressful for Charlene, and when her mom woke her up and started nagging her in the morning, she felt overwhelmed by her mom's pressure. The challenge was that it affected the family being on time for school and impacted the morning's mood and atmosphere. By the time everyone got to school, Charlene and her mom were both exhausted, and *the day had just started.*

Charlene's sensitivity was with the feeling of the clothes on her skin. Her mom was frustrated because she had bought Charlene lots of new clothes for school, but Charlene felt that they all were uncomfortable. Charlene's physical response went from nothing to full-blown anger in only a short period every morning. How could we get Charlene to recognize what made her angry and learn how to control her emotions?

Self-Regulation

The ability to manage stress and control emotions is known as self-regulation. Self-regulation is when we learn how to identify the stressors and learn ways to bring the stress response we are experiencing into a manageable and tolerable state.[20]

For some children, they may need help to learn how to self-regulate or find the balance. Dr. Shanker, in his book *Self-Reg,*[20] identified a five-step approach to finding balance or self-regulation. The first is being able to determine when a child is overstressed. Because everyone's stress response is different, this is crucial in knowing when to investigate further. It is not just a child who is throwing tantrums who is overstressed; it could also be a child who is inattentive, disengaged, and withdrawn. There could be a multiplier effect of numerous stressors on a person's life at the same time. You can notice the multiplier effect when your emotions change depending on what else is going on at that moment. People are generally more irritable when they are tired or hungry or had a bad day. You may tolerate a song on the radio in the morning on the way to work, but on the way home, when you are tired, it may make you irritable.[20]

Once you identify that a child is overstressed, the second step is to spend the time with them to determine what is causing the stress.[20] It is essential at this point to understand the child's whole story. Stress can be from one moment or an accumulation of what a child is exposed to from the caregiver—their sense of belonging, sensory responses, and learning needs. This brings us back to the topics the last few chapters covered. All the unique characteristics you discovered about a child will give you clues into what is triggering the stress and can be key to recognizing how to help a child.

Once you understand the stress, self-regulation moves into the phase of removing or reducing the stress. If you are at a concert and the music is blaring, and you feel overwhelmed by the noise, it will be hard to move into self-regulation or find a sense of calm unless you leave the concert first. Leaving the concert may not get your heart rate down and may not increase your focus yet, but it eliminates the stresses that your body can't handle anymore. In Charlene's case, she was overstressed because of her clothing choices in the morning, and her stress was amplified by her mom waking her up and nagging. By taking that fight away and allowing her to wear only the clothes that she could tolerate, her stressors were decreased.[20]

According to Dr. Shanker, the fourth step is to recognize those times that you are becoming overstressed.[20] Sometimes, if we know what the stressors are, we can actively avoid them. Other times, we may be in a situation that is causing us stress, and we need to become aware of how we are feeling. This self-awareness step is critical because if we can't acknowledge that we are becoming stressed, we won't take the actionable steps to change our state.

Can you think of a time that you were feeling overwhelmed and what made you feel that way?

You may know that feeling. When you feel overwhelmed, you may have trouble focusing, and you may become anxious. Was it one activity, or a thought, or was it an accumulation of many things that made it feel overwhelming, such as that multiplier effect? You check in with yourself to see if you are hungry, thirsty, or tired. You might shift your weight or change positions. You may look around and see what else is going on that could be affecting you. Adults often can recognize that something doesn't feel right and then make changes. Children often don't realize when they are overstressed, or if they do, they may have difficulty communicating, as they haven't yet developed the language to express their feelings.

Instead, this is when you may see a child hide under a desk in a classroom, run away, or simply stare out the window. If we are not in tune with the child, we may miss what a child is trying to tell us. Since each child is unique, there can be a group of children in the same classroom, and each child will have a different experience. It is about perspective. Look at the experience from the perspective of each child, instead of your viewpoint. Then, when a child feels overwhelmed and stressed, acknowledge their feelings, as they are valid for them, and then figure out what they need in this situation, not what you need.

According to Dr. Shanker, the last step is helping children learn how to respond when they feel stressed or overwhelmed and help them to find their sense of calm or balance.[20] I discussed earlier the different answers I received when I asked a group of parents this same question:

What did you do to feel less overwhelmed?

For each of us, this answer will be different. That is the key. Different. With good intention, people often try to impose activities on others because it helps them get calm. Yet, these same activities can have a negative or opposite effect on others. This is why it is called self-regulation. The emphasis is on what works for the self, not just regulation techniques. Deep breathing may make a child anxious, or chime bells may cause a child to act out. It will come down to what works for each child, which will be as unique as the child is. Teaching children this process of learning self-regulation can feel stressful, but it is essential to find a healthy strategy that works for them to find calm in the world, as it will set them up for success when everything feels overwhelming.

Teaching Children How to Recognize Feelings

Much of the information we have covered so far in this chapter refers to abstract feelings. Connecting this language to a child's understanding can be difficult. It is not easy to get a child to recognize their feelings, especially when, as discussed before, the part of their brain that regulates self-control, reasoning, and emotions may not be fully functioning yet. For a child, using words like "calm down" or "relax" may also not mean anything, especially if they don't understand abstract words. Even words like "you look mad" or "I think you're angry" when a child is visibly upset is telling a child how they feel instead of asking them how they are feeling.

Teaching children how to bring language to their feelings can be crucial in unlocking some of their frustration. It then opens up communication with the caregivers to understand how a child is feeling. Teaching this process with a child involves many child–caregiver interactions that can reiterate the ideas in their daily lives. The goal is to repeatedly expose a child to the same kind of information and language, creating brain pathways that connect the feelings to what we should do. We can't just tell a child to "use their words" when they may not have the words to use. As this is a learning process of a new skill, it is essential to ensure the readiness to learn discussed in Chapter 6, including ensuring the child is in a calm or balanced state. *Not when they are overstressed or withdrawn.*

One way to teach the language around feelings and self-regulation is through an occupational therapy program designed by Mary Sue Williams, OTR/L, and Sherry Shellenberger, OTR/L, called the Alert Program®.[23] A program like the Alert Program® tries to bring the language to a place where children can understand it. It focuses on self-regulation by comparing our feelings to the engine of a car. When an engine goes into high gear, we feel overwhelmed and anxious, and when our engine is in low gear, we are at low energy or withdrawn. When our engine is just right, we can be focused and attentive. Using the concept of an engine in high gear, low gear, and just right will work for some children.[23] Others may relate more to the analogy that the gas tank is empty or full, or compare the feelings to animals or a program called the Zones of Regulations™, which shows the growing stress as related to different colors.[24]

Even using this terminology, many children will have difficulty connecting the words to their emotions. A practical method is first to learn how to describe how other people may be experiencing different emotions by looking at pictures or videos. Social stories are an example of a sequence of images that describe actual steps in a real-life event. Social stories come from the idea that we can identify and describe what happens to other people and decide what choices they should make external to us. Children who are concrete learners or need structure and order can often describe cause and effect in others. Therefore, you can discuss feelings by looking at pictures and use the language you have chosen to identify how the person in the image may be feeling. An example of a picture sequence would involve a child playing with a toy and someone takes his toy. The child was then angry and crying. This sequence describes the emotions that may be associated with this event. Say we named the child in the picture Johnny. Johnny just lost his toy, and he is angry. His engine is now in high gear.[23]

Another method that often works with children is to do role-playing or pretend play. In this method, a child can engage in active participation with others to think about what it may feel like if you had your favorite toy and someone took it. In this instance, because it is pretend play, the child knows that someone will take his toy, so the emotion will just be described and not felt.

Also, if an adult uses this language when we describe how we are feeling personally with a child, a child will be able to see it in action and understand what your reaction is. I know when I am stressed, but instead of just dealing with it independently, I can be vocal and say to my kids that my engine is running on high right now.[23] Adding in what I would do, such as I am going to have a cup of tea or go for a walk, will teach them the whole cycle and model positive behavior. It would be different if I picked up my phone and disengaged, as this would not reflect a positive behavior, as often social media can be triggering of other feelings. Likewise, it would help to tell the child your engine is in low gear when you don't have enough energy and how you would react in this instance.[23]

By using these teaching methods, you are creating connections in a child's brain between words, actions, and emotions. Teaching them to recognize the feelings in other people can then transfer to recognizing the feelings within themselves. If a child is upset, you can now relate it to pictures you saw and reframe the conversation to be relatable, such as "Do you feel angry and mad like Johnny did?" Adding in the words related to the engine analogy, you could say, "Is your engine in high gear?"[23]

Beyond helping a child understand when they feel overwhelmed, they also need to learn what makes a child feel calm and safe. What activities do they like to do? What helps them to relax?

Finding the "Just Right" State

Sometimes, children don't know what makes them feel "just right" or calm. A parent or guardian may have clues into the activities that a child enjoys. It is essential to start with understanding a child's sensory preferences. In Chapter 5, we discussed sensory activities to help calm a child. A child tends to gravitate towards or crave what will be more aligned with what makes them feel calmer. It is then a process of exposure to different activities that can identify someone's preferences. This can be done by checking in with a child after doing an activity to see how it made them feel. A child may enjoy listening to sounds, but may become anxious if there is a violin in the music or if the bass is too strong. Therefore, the wrong sound may have a negative impact on what you are trying to accomplish. It doesn't mean that all sounds are wrong; you need to investigate further what works.

As an adult, you would have to be a detective and try to figure out what it is between the different sounds to understand what may be less appealing to a child. A child who craves chewing on things may find chewing necklaces satisfying, but may find pretzels not helping, as that action leaves a dry feeling in the mouth. Going through different activities should happen over time, and it is not recommended to be done all at once. The key is to keep an ongoing record of what you discover has a calming effect. The goal is to create a playbook or toolkit of suggested activities that help a child find calm. When they are overstimulated, presenting them with something they have already chosen that they enjoy is much more useful than working through this process when their engines are high.

For some children with multiple sensory cravings, using a sensory room can be a go-to to help a child find that balance if the child has access to one. The sensory room often provides auditory, visual, tactile, and vestibular activities that can be calming to a child. It may not be the right place for all children to go. Often, a sensory room can be recommended by an occupational therapist, if it is appropriate for a student. It needs to be a place that helps the child find balance and not overstimulate them to the point that they leave there feeling more irritable than when they got there.

You can also gain some ideas by again using the pictures we discussed earlier and seeing how others find their balanced state. You can even watch part of a movie or a television show. In the show, there is often a point where the actors display times of relaxation, such as sitting near a fire, snuggled on a couch with a hot chocolate, petting a dog, taking a bath. These activities let the viewer get the sense that at that moment, that character is calm.

Charlene knew that her clothing made her engine run high. Her mom waking her up loudly and nagging at her was too much to handle in the morning. Charlene was 10 years old, so we talked about what kinds of activities she liked to do when she was at home and how they made her feel. Through our discussion, it was clear that Charlene enjoyed listening to music and coloring. She also knew what clothing she could wear that she could tolerate, *although socks were out of the question.*

Finding Charlene's balance helped her understand her sensory needs and make accommodations to choose clothes that she felt comfortable in. We were also able to identify that she can put some music on and do some coloring for a few minutes to help her body get back to its balanced state when she is starting to feel overwhelmed. Allowing her to be a part of this decision helped her be aware of what she needed to do if she felt like her engine was running on high. From this experience, Charlene also learned that if she felt overwhelmed during the day, she could always go back to listening to music, which brought her into that calmer state.

Sam was a child discussed in a previous chapter who was overwhelmed with the classroom noises. He had difficulty with his communication skills and would become frustrated. His stressor was the classroom noises, so if we stayed in the classroom and worked on coloring or some other activity he enjoyed, it would not help him find his balance. Those activities will only work when the stressors have been removed. By taking Sam out of the classroom to the hallway or to a quiet room and working on an activity that he enjoyed, Sam was able to self-regulate. Each time we left, we would first point to a symbol on his desk that meant hallway. Teaching Sam how to recognize that it was too much in the classroom was the key to making him aware of how to self-regulate.

As someone working with children, it is important to set a good example of how we self-regulate. Try to reflect on your ability to regulate your emotions and recognize the different emotional states you may be in. What if you spend most of your day running behind, always stressed, and not able to take a break? Not only are you going to run out of energy at some point, but you are also not going to be able to demonstrate what it means to self-regulate. When children can see us take time for ourselves, do some deep breathing, have a cup of tea, have a snack, go for a walk, or do some mindfulness minutes, they can begin to get a sense of what self-regulation looks like.

The same can be said for those days where you don't have enough energy even to get up and start an activity. If a child sees you unmotivated and withdrawn, what will they learn from watching you? Being overstimulated or in high stress is one extreme, but when you are under-stimulated and low energy, that is the other extreme. Suppose a child can see that when we don't feel very motivated, we do activities such as take a walk or listen to some energetic music that increases our energy. In that case, it will help them learn that these activities work on both sides of the spectrum.

Purposefully Practicing Self-Regulation Daily

How do you get a child to identify that they need to do some self-regulation activities daily? Regularly doing check-ins to see how their engine is running or how they are feeling is important for us to begin to become aware of how they feel at specific moments. Using the same language consistently every day is essential to build the connections within a child's brain.[23]

This is the same process for building any form of a routine or independence with a child. If you are trying to teach a child to get dressed independently, you would first connect the language of getting dressed to clothing images. The sequence of getting clothes on needs to be the same each time so the brain can begin to recognize the patterns of getting dressed. For instance, if one day you put underwear on your child, then pants, and then the shirt, but on the next day you start with the shirt, and then underwear, and then pants, the organization of that information is now not creating a consistent pathway in the child's brain to remember the sequence.

If it is part of the routine to check in and see how someone feels, it is less irritable for a child than to only point out when they need to calm down. Integrating this into a group setting or a classroom routine can make it more normal to check in with yourself and how you feel. Sometimes, kids need some prompting or visual cues. From color charts to faces on a spectrum to numbers, there are many strategies that can help children identify how they are feeling. Once a child can identify this, you would allow them to do an activity and then re-evaluate if they feel any different.

At a workplace, I have heard from people who have mental health check-ins daily during their team meetings. It creates the space and conversation to identify where you are at and what you need to help you get to where you want to be. It decreases the stigma or focus around only identifying those that are struggling, and it recognizes that we all need to be aware of our feelings.

If someone came up to me and said, "You seem mad," it would make me even angrier. If someone checked in daily and instead asked, "How are you feeling today," it would open up that opportunity to be self-reflective.

Sam began to understand when he was overwhelmed in the classroom. Because previously, when we left the classroom, we would point to a picture of the hallway, Sam started to independently use the symbol on his desk that identified that he wanted to go for a walk. It was through the daily repetition that he built the brain pathway to know that hallway meant calm. It was a massive step for him to recognize the need to remove the stressors and allow him to have a break.

Self-regulation is an active process. Once we get into a neutral state, it may only take a look in the wrong direction to trigger another response. If a child can become aware of what creates that response, they can learn to avoid those interactions over time.

Why Can't We All Do the Same Activity?

Each child is unique and has their own story of who they are. At the beginning of this chapter, when I asked the parent group what they do to help them get into a calm state, they all responded with different activities.

I know that if I were to go out and garden, I would not be calm. Me and gardens do not get along. I was so stressed working in a garden when I was pregnant, it actually put me into labor. Yet, for others, the time in nature, picking away at the weeds, is relaxing and releasing. For others, baths were not something they enjoyed.

So why is this?

It can go back to the sensory preferences that we covered in Chapter 5. The way that we process the sensory information in our brains is different for each person. The smells, sounds, textures, tastes, or movement elicits a heightened response, a neutral response, or a calming response. Often, children crave sensory input because this input makes them feel more relaxed or calmer.

Think about a child who will stay on the swing for half an hour if they could. This child craves the vestibular input of swings or spinning. If this child was asked to sit in an assembly at school for an hour with their legs crossed, they might last only 10 minutes before they start fidgeting and eventually disrupt others. If forced to stay in the assembly, you might find their misbehavior increases to the point that the child is removed and may be penalized for their actions. Instead, the child's teacher or caregiver needed to recognize that this child would need to have some movement again to help them find their calm. If you knew that this was something a child struggled with, setting them up for success would look like allowing them to sit on a bouncing recliner chair in the gym during assembly; that way, they could move while they listened.

This type of movement may not work for someone with gravitational insecurities. It may be the movement that is the stressor for them. For this child, figuring out what is calming for them will look different. Often, children with gravitational insecurity enjoy playing with toys while lying on the ground. It is one of the most stable positions, and then they don't need to worry about controlling their body in space. Setting this child up for success would be to give them time to transition their movements from one space to another and set them to transition to lying down if they needed to find that sense of calm.

One method did not work for both children because their sensory needs were different. Again, this is why it is called self-regulation. Each person will have their own needs.

Sometimes, the activities also don't work if the child is so overstimulated that their brain is only in survival mode. It can be because of the multiplier effect, as referred to by Dr. Shanker.[20] At this point, removing all stressors and allowing some time to pass will help them be able to come to the point that you can introduce one of their calming activities.

When the recommendation or the choice is the caregiver's and not the child's, this can also influence its effectiveness. For instance, demanding a child go outside and play if they are stressed may only aggravate them further. Although it may be with the best intentions, your approach is coming from a control approach that does not acknowledge the child's feelings at all. Instead, as Dr. Greene discussed in his book, using the Plan B approach involves working with the child to develop a mutually agreed-upon solution.[22] By including the child in the process, you help them learn how to become active participants in their self-regulation. It often takes some extra time, but the connection you will have built with the child will affect their sense of belonging and significance. This will set the framework for increased active participation in other activities.[9]

Why Does It Work This Time, But Doesn't the Next Time?

Learning what strategies are effective for self-regulation is valuable, as it can create a playbook or toolbox with lots of different ideas. It is exciting to find something that works effectively to help balance a child or even for ourselves. What can be frustrating is when those strategies or activities stop working.

I used to wake up at 6:30 am every morning. As soon as I heard my alarm, I would jump out of bed and start my day. Over time, I would hear my alarm less and less. Did my alarm change at all? No, but my brain's reactivity to it became less.

The same can happen to activities we do. When the effectiveness wears off, it is important to try something different or re-evaluate what that activity is trying to accomplish. It is also why it is valuable to have a toolbox full of various activities or suggestions so that the variety of the activities will keep the body engaged.

Although simplified to help understand the general process of self-regulation, the ideas that I covered in this chapter offer the same approach to help a child, teen, or adult find ways to self-regulate. In the teenage and adult years, we can recognize our stressors, which may be heightened by hormones, but we may find unhealthy ways of self-regulating. Taking the same approach of understanding what the stressor entails, recognizing what activities help self-regulate you, and then creating the environment that encourages and promotes opportunities for these activities to happen will help you find balance. If the environment we are in is conducive to our sensory and learning needs, it can help us be more productive and engaged. This next chapter will identify key ways to assess and modify the environment to meet those needs.

Chapter Reflections

1. What does it mean to self-regulate?
2. Why is it important to first be able to identify that you are stressed?
3. Why is it important to eliminate the stressor before you self-regulate?
4. Why is important to find the "just right" state?
5. Why don't the same calming activities work for all of us?

9 Integrating Into the Environment

The setting of a child's story can make a large impact on how a child reacts. Since the environment is constantly changing, learning to find a sense of balance in the world can be a big task for some people, especially children. Up to this point in the book, the focus has been mainly inwards and understanding what makes the child's story unique. What I haven't focused on a great deal is how different environments can affect each story. The elements that create each environment may impact how a child will function within each location. It is more than what we see or touch that makes up the environment.

Think about your home. Consider the physical structure of the walls, doors, and windows, the furniture within it, and the decorative touches that make it your own. Your home can also be shared with others who add their own touches and personalities. It can be a place of joy and happiness or sadness and fear. It can be a place that follows traditions passed down from generations before you, good or not so good, and contains rules spoken or unspoken that need to be followed. Your home environment is more than just your physical address.

A bus is also an environment. It is much different from a house, but contains similar elements. Children ride buses to school every day. One boy I worked with struggled with getting on the bus. He would scream when he had to get on the school bus in the morning. Despite his love for buses, he could not handle the way the environment made him feel. Just like a home, the bus has windows and doors and furniture. Different people share the space, and there are rules that need to be followed.

Think about how many more environments you navigate in one single day.

Many people think it could be an easy adaptation for a child with unique needs, but modifying the environment is complex, and many parts are out of our control. Understanding how to create, plan, and prepare to navigate the world using the information we have is key to helping a child reach their potential.

What Makes Up an Environment?

The term environment is defined as anything that is outside of us and can create a response from us.[4] It means that any space where a child needs to process

DOI: 10.4324/9781003166405-9

or engage in is their environment. Their experience in this space will relate to their physical needs and sensory preferences, sense of belonging, and ability to learn.

As outlined in Chapter 2, I used the CMOP-E as a guiding model for this book. You might want to refer back to Figure 2.1 in Chapter 2. The environment within this model is divided into four main elements: physical, social, institutional, and cultural.[4] The environment is like a cake. We only see the outside icing of the cake, but there is a lot inside that makes up the space.

The physical elements are what we see. It is the icing on the cake. It includes all the physical buildings, vehicles, outdoor spaces, technology, and any other tangible materials that a child will encounter. It could consist of home, school, cars, buses, community centers, arenas, parks, playgrounds, gaming systems, and computers, to name only a few.

The physical elements include the specifics within each space, including the sensory experiences that they create. As adults, we may not even notice the sensory inputs we are receiving, as our brains have become accustomed to them and no longer trigger any reaction. From the lights on the ceiling to the wind's sound on the windows, it is essential to become more aware of each environment's sensory experiences. This is because these inputs can still impact some people. When working with children, we need to recognize how children's sensory preferences will tolerate a space, or if they will need some accommodations made to help them. It is valuable to train your brain to focus on one sense at a time as you enter a physical space and take note of what you notice.

Take a moment and go stand in your bedroom and listen to the noises you make walking around, opening and closing drawers, doors, and curtains. Now go into the bathroom and do the same, but add flushing the toilet, running the water, and turning on the fan. The space in your bedroom is often quieter because of the bed and carpet that dampen the sound. The bathroom is often tile, glass, and ceramics. The sounds in a bathroom will echo differently than the sounds in a bedroom. You may not have noticed the sounds anymore, as your sensory system has become accustomed to them. Yet, for someone hyper-sensitive to sound, the noises in a bathroom can be overwhelming and may affect their willingness to use the bathroom or shower, and that *is just focusing on the sound.*

Do the same activity, but now focus on the things you touch and notice the texture and temperature. What do you feel? The softness of the mattress on a bed or the roughness of the carpet in the bedroom. Is the bathroom tile cold? Is the toilet seat hard and cold? Are the towels damp or dry?

Now be aware of the smells. The smells of the bedroom are often the familiar smell of the clothes you wear, the bed you sleep in. On the other hand, the bathroom can often smell of cleaner, toothpaste, or human waste if someone just went to the bathroom.

As you go through each of the sensory systems, you can see how much our brain needs to process to move throughout the physical elements, and *that was just within a house.* Think about all the spaces within a school: the gym, cafeteria, washrooms with multiple toilets, classrooms, hallways, libraries, and music rooms. Within each of these spaces, the feelings, sounds, and smells that a child might experience will be different. Vehicles such as a car or a bus include a moving component that challenges our vestibular system. Even the space outdoors with the unique sounds, smells, and uneven ground can affect our proprioceptive system. Can you see why some children may want to stay in one space that they feel comfortable in, or how children who have difficulty processing sensory inputs are already running their engines on "high gear" when they leave their home?

Each physical space a child may encounter needs to be evaluated from the perspective of the child's sensory preferences. As you become more mindful of the sensory experience, it becomes more apparent how the environment's physical elements may affect them.

The inside of the cake is made up of the next three elements of the environment. One layer is the social elements of the environment. The social elements include all the people who are located within the space that you are in. In the home environment, the people would consist of family members who live at the house and friends and relatives who visit. At school, it would include all the students in the class, the teachers, kids on the playground, and support staff at the school. Each environment will have different social elements, including how people are expected to engage and act and also their role in the environment. As we discussed at the beginning of the book, each person within that space will have their own physical needs, sensory preferences, learning styles, past experiences, and behaviors. Each person's mood and emotions will be different depending on the moment. Matching sensory preferences amongst a social environment is often challenging. That is why people tend to gravitate towards common interest groups where they can relate to others more easily.

Luca was a boy in a class who was hypersensitive to sounds. He had difficulty concentrating when there were other sounds around. Luca was also a concrete thinker. He knew the rules, and rules were meant to be followed. Ethan was another boy in Luca's class. Ethan had difficulty focusing in class and would often get anxious over missing information. Ethan's self-regulation method was to hum to himself because the vibrations from the humming were calming to Ethan. Ethan was seated right next to Luca in class, which created a challenging environment for Luca to concentrate, as Ethan was often humming. Luca was upset because no one was supposed to make noise while the teacher was talking. Because Ethan was humming, both of them missed the information in class. The social elements of this environment made it challenging for both children to fully participate in the class. Even the modifications to the environment for each child may not take into account the social elements of the people around them. Yet these social elements can have a significant impact on a child.

Sometimes, the differing roles of the people in the environment can also impact a child's ability to manage the environment. Ethan did better with having a specific educational assistant (EA) with him one-on-one at school. When Ethan's EA was present, Ethan would be less anxious because he knew that someone was there to help if he needed it, and he had a special relationship with this EA. He would decrease his humming because having the emotional support of someone was important for Ethan to function in this environment.

Remember, these are only two children from a class of often 20–30 children. Each child may have their own needs. Think about all the people in a church, a grocery store, or a shopping mall. Although you may not interact directly, the movement, sound, smell, and sight of the people in these environments can be overstimulating to some and enjoyable for others.

Another cake layer is the institutional elements. These are the rules, policies, and practices that govern any environment and are specific to that space's expectations. It could include government, churches, schools, sports teams, and clubs, and there often are even rules within a home. The institutional elements can impact the engagement of children within these environments. The education system is an example of practices built many years ago during the industrial revolution. The concept of learning at desks and chairs for six to seven hours per day was meant to prepare workers to work in factories. Although the curriculum has changed, using a curriculum as a guiding practice has not. It requires all children to keep up with the set expectations based on generalized assumptions of children's abilities. The requirement for testing, grades, and assignments can induce anxiety in children who struggle with learning. If children are behind in these expectations, is it the child's learning capacity or is it the lack of flexibility in the curriculum's practices? There are also the intertwined government regulations that influence the education system, creating an environment that may or may not match the learning needs of the children it serves. It can be challenging to change the current practices. Therefore, it is essential to understand their existence and how they apply to a child.

Nya had difficulty staying in her seat. Like many, she was required to stay at her desk sitting on the hard chair in her class. Nya would always wiggle and move, and it would often become so uncomfortable for her that she would get up and walk around. She would sharpen her pencil, throw something in the garbage, or wander pretending she was looking for something. The teacher wanted the children to stay at their desks to not distract others, so Nya would repeatedly be asked to return to her desk. Nya knew that the only other reason she was allowed to get up was to go to the bathroom. She would raise her hand and go to the bathroom almost every hour. It became such an issue that the teacher called Nya's parents to ask them if she should see a doctor because of the number of times she went. The challenge was: Nya never really had to go to the bathroom, but she was otherwise stuck staying at her desk because of the expectations of the classroom. It was her way of self-regulating her body because she needed to move to focus. If she asked if she could go for a walk, she would not be allowed, as safety policies prohibited students from wandering the hallways unattended unless they had to go to the bathroom or had a staff member with them.

I have also worked with children similar to Nya, whose requests to use the bathroom were denied by the teacher, and so the child began acting out so that they would be sent to the principal's office so that they could get out of class. When the rules of the environment don't match the child's needs, we can see the outward displays of behaviors.

Rules can also be useful for some children, especially those who like to know what to expect. Children may thrive on schedules and routines, even though others resist the confines of any structure. Luca was a child who wanted rules, structure, and order. His teacher had posted the schedule for the week on the wall, and Luca felt comfort in knowing what was going to happen next. He also liked to know what was expected of him. The rules of how to act made it clear to him what he should be doing. What was frustrating to him was when others did not follow the rules of the class. When people didn't raise their hand to speak or got out of their desk without asking, it made Luca angry. Luca was a very concrete thinker and knew that rules were to be followed. Luca's challenge was that he struggled with being flexible when the schedule would change, a new teacher would fill in when his teacher was sick, or when rules were broken or ignored.

In Chapter 7 on behaviors, we talked about a girl named Ramona who was in Grade 9. Because of her family experiences, she struggled with authority and being bound by rules. An environment like school would make it challenging for her to succeed.

The last layer of the cake consists of the cultural elements of the environment. Cultural elements are those practices and traditions associated with a group, religion, or culture. The incorporation of religion in schools is an example of cultural elements that affect the school's daily activities. Singing of the national anthem, celebrating holidays, and having family meals are all examples of cultural traditions. They can create some comfort and routines in family life and invoke a more profound sense of connection and belonging amongst families and groups.

Cultural upbringing can also play into how someone interacts with the environment. In Chapter 2 of this book, I discussed a mom who never taught her child how to use toilet paper, as it was their practice to take baths or use warm washcloths. This practice affected the child's experience at school, as he was not comfortable going to the washroom.

Many of the environments that a child will engage in will have all four elements, such as the home and bus example at the beginning of this chapter. A school also has specific physical spaces, the interaction of many different people, a set of governing principles and rules, and the cultural influences of the community or religious affiliation it represents. Some factors can change or be modified in each of these elements, but there are lots that we cannot always control.

Assessing a Child's Environment

As we have covered so far in this chapter, there are many different elements of the environment. The way a child perceives, understands, and functions within the space will depend on how their brain interprets the information. As a caregiver or someone working with a child, it is important to go back to what we keep reviewing—understanding the history, sensory preferences, and learning needs first. Scanning the environment using each of our senses is a valuable way to start. Always return to the child's perspective. Focus on what a child would see, smell, hear, and touch and how they would move about the area on an average day. Then when a child is overwhelmed, notice if anything has changed in the environment. It will give us clues to understand what elements are overwhelming to the child. Then repeat this in every environment that they will engage in. Educating and engaging other caregivers in this process will be important, as often, there are different people present with the child. Remember that our personal preferences will be very different from the child's, so what does not affect you or I may significantly affect the child.

In my practice, I spend a lot of time educating parents or caregivers on the child's needs and recognizing and assessing the environment based on those needs. The parents are often present or involved in more than one environment and can express their child's needs and preferences to others. This becomes part of the child's story, and if done effectively, as we will cover in a later chapter, it can create the consistency children often need.

What You Can Control

Within any environment, there are often only a few things that we can control. In some spaces, we can control what physical elements are present, the routines and schedules, the equipment a child can use or have with them, and sometimes control who is present. These suggestions are by no means inclusive, but the knowledge of what you can and can't control highlights how much a child still needs to process at any given time.

By starting with a space conducive to their needs, we can set a child up with equipment that we know may help them. The easiest way to start is by changing or modifying any of the physical elements in the space. These objects can provide comfort and security because they can be modified to fit the child's needs. An excellent place to start is where a child sleeps or a child's bedroom. It is a space in the home that, when everything else may become overwhelming, they can go to. When a child can calm their body, they can more easily calm their mind. Using night lights, the right type of comforter, a supportive chair, or a fitted desk are all ways to modify their bedroom. A parent may add a relaxing scent to help soothe a child who may be sensitive to smells or play music when a child goes to bed to create a sense of calm.

Other spaces within the home where a child may need to participate or focus on a task may benefit from consistent equipment. If a child is easily distracted or struggles with attention, a cluttered or disorganized house can affect them without you even realizing it. The disorganization and clutter force their eyes to move from space to space and force their brains to think about many different things. Eliminating clutter in some instances can help a child find that sense of calm.

If eating is difficult for a child, creating a space that eliminates any of the extra sensory inputs that bother a child can help them work on eating. Look at the chair the child is sitting on. If they find the chair too firm, can you put a cushion on it, or can the child stand while eating? Can you turn off any noises in the house? What cutlery can you change? I have worked with children who can't eat because of the sound of others chewing or using cutlery on their plates. In this case, consider using plastic forks instead of metal forks, as the sound is very different.

It can be more challenging to set up a shared environment like a classroom, especially if a child is sensitive to lights, sounds, and movement. In a school, there are few things you can control. Yet if you can create a physical spot in the classroom that can eliminate as much stimulation as possible, it will make it easier for the child to function. Can they be at the front of the classroom? Are the walls bare in front of them? Can you put tennis balls on the feet of all the chairs to decrease the chairs' sounds on the floor? Can the light be lowered when the teacher is teaching, especially if the windows can let in the natural light? Can the child wear headphones that limit the sound or are connected to an FM system that the teacher wears? These are the kinds of accommodations that can help you to try and create the environment that the child needs within a larger setting just by making a few minor changes.

Within the school, can you also integrate a space that is calming for a child? For example, adding a tent or playhouse allows the child somewhere to go away from lights and people or add a swing or trampoline inside to create an area that is safe for vestibular movement.

It is also valuable to create consistencies in other aspects of the environment. The use of consistent routines and schedules can create comfort for children, as the repetition allows them to build the brain's pathways, and it becomes something that they recognize. The same pattern of behavior becomes automatic. In a home, it can be the schedule from when they wake up to leave for school, or in the classroom, it can be the day's schedule for subjects and breaks. Visually displaying these schedules in places that a child can refer to is another consistent part, ensuring that the routines and schedules are followed. The use of consistent language such as "1–2–3, eyes on me" creates a calm trigger to change the focus and attention back onto the teacher.

If we can't control the whole environment, we can prepare a child with equipment to function in an environment to create a more productive and positive space. I did this for the boy who struggled with the bus because of the sound. Once we determined why he was overwhelmed, I provided him with noise-canceling headphones that he could use whenever he was in a space that had the sound that bothered him. His anxiety decreased for going to the bus and getting on the bus. Some families have headphones that they leave in the car that help with any social outing like a grocery store or shopping mall. We can't change these environments' sounds, but we can lessen the exposure to the sounds that they may experience. Integrating other equipment at school, such as having access to computers or tablets, can decrease school anxieties when it comes to learning or assignments.

The same can be said about a consistent caregiver or support worker at school. When a child creates a bond with someone, that bond increases their sense of belonging and safety—seeing the same person every day can be comforting. There is often a significant difference in a child's behaviors when their support worker or teacher is not at school for a day.

The challenge is that we can't control all aspects of the environment. So, giving a child equipment, schedules, and places that they can consistently turn to will bring that sense of control when their world feels out of control.

Preparing a Child for the Elements They Can't Control

For the elements that we can't control in the environment, it is essential to plan how a child will navigate these. Preparing a child, setting expectations, and slowly building tolerance are all strategies that can help a child learn how to navigate an uncontrollable environment.

The kitchen is an excellent example of an environment that is changing. The sound and smells of cooking food will change daily. The kitchen can have music playing in the background, fan's on, and food is cooking on the stovetop, all of which can be heard and smelled.

If you walked into this environment and weren't expecting it, you could feel overwhelmed, especially if you are sensitive to sounds and smells. What can help is to communicate or prepare a child for what will happen in the future, letting those around know there will be cooking going on in the kitchen, the fan will be on, and they may smell the food. By preparing the brain that this will happen, you can take away the surprise element that can trigger overwhelm.

Similarly, if you are going to the grocery store, you can prepare a child for what they might encounter. As adults, we can often predict the general experiences in different settings. For example, a grocery store will have bright lights, noisy carts, lots of people, and overhead announcements. We may not know how these will impact the child exactly, but we can use our insight to help the child prepare for the experience using some of their self-regulation skills we reviewed in Chapter 8. Once in the environment, we need to check in often with how they feel to get a sense of their tolerance. When a child feels overwhelmed or stressed, you can implement one of their self-regulation strategies or return to a more controlled environment.

Part of being prepared is also knowing what the expectations are. It is very similar to a parenting method that I learned when I first became a parent. If we communicate expectations with a child before an activity, event, or space, children can plan to the best of their ability to act based on the expectations. Before we go into a toy store to buy one of their friends a toy for their birthday, I sit in the car with my children and discuss why we are at the toy store and who we are buying a gift for, acknowledge that there are lots of nice toys at the store, but we are only buying a gift for the friend. It has now set the expectations for what we are going to do at the store. When you are in the store, instead of just saying no to the child, you can now remind them about the conversation in the car. They now share ownership over the plan for the visit to the store.

The same technique can be used with a child before any activity they are participating in. Communicating the plan and expectation before the activity is like giving your brain a preview of the movie. It is helping your brain to connect to those learning hooks that we discussed in Chapter 6. The brain is more prepared because you have them thinking about what they need before getting into a space and the potential for overwhelm.

Building up a tolerance is another good strategy for environments that you can't control. Start with smaller pieces of your bigger goal. If a child is learning to be around other people, start with a small group and increase it as they feel comfortable. For example, taking a child to a smaller store with fewer people may be better to start with than going to a crowded mall.

At the beginning of this chapter, I asked you to think about walking into the bathroom. We discussed all the sounds in the bathroom and how overwhelming that can be. Exposing a child to small increments in a space like this will help to build a tolerance, such as walking in and turning on and off the tap until they feel comfortable with this. Then work on turning the tap on and off and touching the water and so on. Similarly, if you are trying to get a child to go to the toilet, start by flushing the toilet, then put toilet paper in the toilet and flush the toilet. Then you build up to the entire task. It is about taking an activity and breaking it down into manageable pieces. Then you work to master each step before adding on another.

As much as we can be proactive and prepare for different environments based on a child's sensory preferences and needs, their emotions and internal body regulation can fluctuate drastically.

Emotions are always changing, and sometimes they can be unrelated to the activity at hand. A child may be in a state of happiness, sadness, fear, anger, and anxiety. Children have a hard time describing their emotions or why they feel this way, but it can impact how they respond to their environment. Acknowledging their feelings and allowing them space to feel that way is essential. Often, it can be a cue that their body is trying to tell them something. Like the sensory triggers we discussed in the last chapter, emotions can tell us that our body is not balanced. These emotional triggers can cause fear or anxiety that will create a ripple effect into the environment that a child used to find calming. Many of the self-regulation techniques discussed in the last chapter will help a child work through these emotional states.

As much as we can plan for and accommodate many sensory systems, the interoception sense or our internal regulation sense is challenging. It is challenging to prepare for when a child is hungry, needs to use the washroom, is tired, or has discomfort. Some children's body systems do not follow the school schedule or the "we are going on a car ride" bathroom visit. Many self-regulation techniques will not work on a child whose body is giving them clues for internal regulation. So, if a child is hungry and goes into a space that is usually calming to them, it won't create that same feeling or the hoped-for result. For example, children who have difficulty focusing just before lunch and can't sit still would not respond well to a sensory room visit, as that will not help their hunger. Likewise, a child who needs to use the bathroom can become angry and violent if they don't fully understand the feeling that their body is trying to tell them about needing to have a bowel movement.

A colleague worked with a child who was non-verbal and was always unsettled in class and would get angry. One day, she took him to the sensory room when he was irritated and kept the light dim to see if he could get back to his "just right" state. Instead, what happened was he fell asleep on the bean bag chair in the room. He was fighting fatigue and didn't know how to express it. She let him sleep for a little bit of the session, and as he slept, she noticed that he was having difficulty with his breathing while he was asleep; it was not rhythmic as it should be. The parents were notified, and when taken to the specialist, he was diagnosed with sleep apnea. His body was so exhausted that his tolerance to do his activities during the day was limited.

There are many moving pieces in an environment. Recognizing that we can't control for all the factors that affect the environment, we just need to acknowledge that these factors exist. Then prepare as much as possible and help a child positively engage in new environments; these will be the building blocks to increase their tolerance.

Choosing the Right Environment for the Task

Remember the story at the beginning of this book about teaching a child how to read on a rollercoaster. The child with their sensory issues would not be very effective at reading because the environment did not match the activity. Changing the environment was essential to match the needs of the child and the activity. Think back to the Person, Environment, and Occupation (PEO)[5] model discussed in Chapter 2. The model described how the person and their needs, the task that you are trying to accomplish, and the environment all need to align for someone to have successful occupational performance.[5]

In this chapter so far, we have outlined the elements that influence an environment. Choosing the right environment for the task is going to make a significant difference in the outcome.

Trying to teach a child how to wash their hands without using a sink and water is not connecting a child to the actual task of washing their hands.

Similarly, if we teach children how to use a fork or spoon, but don't use real food, it can again not connect with the task at hand.

We need to create connections and routines in the environment in which the task will occur: for example, practicing dressing skills in the bedroom and bathroom skills in the bathroom.

In therapy, we try to build up the required skills for an activity by breaking it down into smaller components. Children who struggle with handwriting may have weak hands, so working to build hand strength is important. Likewise, teaching children how to do up buttons and zippers is a precursor for independent dressing. We use swings to work on vestibular skills. When we look for the transfer of the skill to the full task, we need to ensure that the person's needs are matched in the right environment for the activity or occupation they are trying to perform. The right environment can significantly impact how a child's body and mind integrate the knowledge into practice. So, whenever you think about the child's needs and what you are trying to accomplish, ensure that you are in the right environment for those needs.

Depending on the child's goals, using outdoor space can integrate many smaller components that can then be transferable indoors. In her book *Balanced and Barefoot*, Angela Hanscom[25] describes how nature provides a better sensory balanced environment. The experience with the sounds, smells, and sights are much more subtle than indoors. The outdoor experience also allows natural movement patterns to incorporate our balance and body awareness, such as leaning over to pick up sticks to build a fort or climbing over fallen trees. This natural playground allows our body to integrate all the different sensory experiences.[25] So if children are struggling inside, often the change of scenery to outdoors can help if the child is trying to learn different skills.

Where Do You Begin?

Every environment will create a different experience. Parents and caregivers often have an idea of which space creates the most stress for a child. Starting at this space can often alleviate the stress for the child and the parent.

> *Is there one environment that increases your stress response greater than other environments?*
> *What is it about this space?*

Steven was sensitive to sounds and lights and had gravitational insecurities. He spent a lot of time at home in his room playing on his tablet while lying on his bed. He was stressed when he had to do his chores or sit at the table for dinner. He was also occasionally overwhelmed at school when it was too loud or if he had gym class, but Steven absolutely could not stand going in the car. It made it hard to get him to school each day and made it difficult to get him to appointments for therapy. Although all three environments had some similar reactions and the suggestion in one could help the other, the environment causing the most stress to both Steven and the family was the car.

The environment of the car would become priority number one to work on. The lessons that a parent learns from this situation will impact all the other situations throughout the day. Yet the relief provided in this one situation will immediately affect the family if strategies are put into place.

Despite our best efforts to create the perfect environment, we cannot always control all the components. Understanding this and acknowledging what can and cannot change will also help you get a sense of the child's reactions to the many different stimuli, both internal and external. When you understand more about the child's story, the next step is to get those around the child on board with the same strategies, goals, and vision. All of the information provided so far is intended to increase awareness of the fact that there is more to a child's story than what you can see by how they behave. When you have knowledge, you gain the power in making changes that can help a child thrive in their environment.

Chapter Reflections

1. What four elements make up the environment?
2. Why is it important to assess the environment from the perspective of the child?
3. What are some aspects of the environment that you can control?
4. What are aspects of the environment you can't control?
5. How do you choose the right environment for a task?

10 Influence of Family/ Caregiver Support

Up until this point, we have looked at a child's story in relative isolation: what makes a child unique and how they navigate the world. We understand that some of a child's story comes from how they were brought up. This was often a result of the caregiver's influence or the person who is working with the child and how that person was raised.

We also know that a child is still dependent on adults in their lives to help them. This is why it is also very important to be aware of the child's current situation. Where does a child spend the majority of their time? Outside of school, the child spends most of their time at home. If something happens at school with a child, who is the first person the school will contact? It always comes back to the person legally responsible. When we look to the parent/caregiver to help with a child, what we need to consider is how willing, able, and capable they are in helping a child reach their goals.

Family involvement is a major key to a child's success, but what if it's not an option. A mom may be struggling with depression and have three children, of which two children have sensory and learning needs, each of whom is having a tough time at school. Therefore, having great ideas and suggestions for educational or therapeutic goals may be valid for the child, but the mom's ability to implement them may be limited, especially when the mom is taxed with caring for the one child and their siblings, each with their own unique struggles.

We know that there can be positive effects of family involvement on school success and social and emotional development. We also know that, sometimes, it is the family that can have adverse effects on a child. It can be a result of the dynamics of the family around them. When I talk about families, I am referring to the people involved in raising a child. Families are often composed of a group of people. The family structure can consist of the child, single parent or caregiver, two parents, siblings, and sometimes extended families. Everything that I have covered in the book this far applies to each of those people as well. They all have their own story that is unfolding—each with their unique sensory preferences, learning needs, love language, and validation needs. The stressors of others can affect a child's stress, and a child can also become the object of stress within a family.

DOI: 10.4324/9781003166405-10

So, when we look at a child's family, we are not just looking at the caregiver and how they can help that child. It can also be how multiple children in the family interact with each other. There can be fighting amongst siblings for parental attention. Another child may have their own needs that require attention. All of this on top of what other priorities the caregiver may have daily.

Parenting is also one of the most challenging jobs a person can have. Parenting is exhausting, and often parents have their own stressors related to parenting. According to Dr. Shanker, there are five fundamental stressors for parents: helping your child learn how to fit in with others, the empathy parents feel for their children, the competitiveness of parenting, navigating the excessive amounts of stressors children face, and finding the right parenting style.[20]

Parenting comes with no training, and as discussed in a previous chapter, it does not come with a handbook or guide on how to navigate each stage or stress of raising a child. Even if there was a book, each child is so unique we would need to have countless volumes of information. When it comes to parenting, people are doing what they know and are comfortable with. Remember the belief that every child would do well if they could. It highlights the understanding that if you lack the skills or resources, you will not be able to do the task that is asked of you.[19] I believe this to be the same for parents. Let's assume that every parent is doing the best they can with the resources and abilities they have at that moment. This includes energy levels and mental health. We are all human beings who are learning each day. Like everything in life, we don't know that we don't know something until we find out we didn't know it. Say that 10 times fast!

I believe that it comes down to a myriad of factors: differing priorities, understanding, experience, education, support, consensus, and mindset.

If parents knew all the ins and outs of dealing with children, it would be easy, and raising children is far from easy. The most important takeaway is that communication and education are key, and we need to understand that there is often more to someone's life than what we see on the surface, and this includes everyone you meet.

Differing Backgrounds and Lifestyle Priorities

When working with parents and families, it is essential to understand what parents and caregivers value the most regarding raising a child. Many of the choices made are based on lifestyle priorities that have developed in the subconscious from childhood. These choices came out of the way we were raised and match how we navigated the world growing up.[9]

Lifestyle priorities, according to Jane Nelson, "represent the decisions you made throughout your life that affect the way you attempt to find a sense of belonging and significance" (p. 236).[9] It is not just children who want to feel that sense of belonging and significance. It is human nature; it affects all of us. When we discussed children's desires to belong and their mistaken goals for achieving that belonging, it is because they are trying to form their priorities. Strangely, what we learn when we are young will affect our adult choices. Yet, when it comes to parenting, these choices can impact our relationships with our children. Lifestyle priorities are divided into four main categories, including comfort, control, pleasing, and superiority. We often have one preference that is stronger than the others, but we can have influence from more than one. Choosing comfort means that you avoid conflict and tension, whereas choosing control prioritizes structure, order, and organization. When pleasing is a priority, you try to make everything fun for everyone around you, yet when superiority is a focus, this means you need to feel that success and importance in each situation.[9]

These subconscious priorities are essential to understand because they can influence the choices we make as adults and influence how we interact with children. A parent who prioritizes comfort or pleasing with their child may avoid creating boundaries that help a child understand how to navigate the world. Whereas, a parent whose priority is superiority or control may make choices focused on very restrictive boundaries and cause children to feel never good enough.[9]

When two parents have differing underlying priorities in life, it can create conflict within a family and how children are raised. Children are learning through adults' priorities, and that is how they are forming their own. Children understand actions more than they understand words.

Pete and Lacey knew they had grown up differently, but once they were married, the plan was to create a new life together and make their own choices and rules. Yet, when it came to having children, they had very different priorities for how their children would behave and act. Pete grew up in a very strict household, where the rules were never meant to be broken, and if they were, you were scared. That fear kept many behaviors in check. Lacey, on the other hand, grew up with a lot more freedom. She made some mistakes as she was growing up, but her parents allowed her to learn from her mistakes and grow from them. She experienced unconditional love and knew, no matter what, her parents were there for her. When Pete and Lacey's children were school-aged, behaviors in their children began to arise. It wasn't just in one child, but in both, and they had different challenges. As described in Chapter 7, many of these behaviors were age-appropriate displays, or sensory overload, or differing learning styles. Pete wanted to set the rules and strictly follow them, maintaining control, and Lacey wanted to take the gentler approach to avoid tension and conflict.

The lack of consistency in parenting styles and priorities between two parents or caregivers can confuse the child. The relationship between the parents can create power struggles, and they can blame each other for their child's behaviors, missing the potential underlying causes, which could be sensory overload. This can take away from the child's understanding of their boundaries or general expectations of behaviors, which is vital in creating that sense of stability and safety.

It is more challenging when a child struggles outside of the home, such as at school. The school brings in the parent to discuss a plan for the child. In the instance of Pete and Lacey, Pete would come down harder on his child and lean towards stricter rules and more forceful punishment because it is what worked for him. On the other hand, Lacey would be more apt to try to come up with a gentler strategy that included encouraging the child to be an active participant in learning from what happened. Without fully being aware of what your lifestyle priorities are, it can be challenging to come to a compromise in a situation.

As mentioned in Chapter 7, Lacey was moving towards a Plan B, as Dr. Greene refers to it when working with her children.[19] She was trying to make them an active participant in creating a plan and understanding of why the behaviors happened and how to effectively self-regulate. On the other hand, Pete was more focused on his plan, which stemmed from control and discipline: "My way or the highway." From the school perspective, having these two parenting styles or priorities, it can be hard to get a consensus on a plan to best help their child.[19] Creating a collaborative conversation will be covered in the next chapter. The first part of the equation is understanding each family member's perspective on a child. What does each of them bring to the conversation from their history, their priorities? What are they most worried about?

Think about your priorities in life. What resonates the most with your lifestyle?

Marco was a boy I worked with who struggled with anxiety and transitions. He was a very concrete learner, meaning that he did not understand abstract words, and he craved lots of vestibular movement. The environmental set up for Marco was vital for helping to keep him balanced and self-regulated. Marco's parents' separation was not a very amicable separation, so there was a lot of tension between them. One parent tried to keep Marco to his schedule and routine and give him the outlets he needed. The other parent wanted Marco to have fun and wanted to let Marco have a break from any of the rigidness of schedules or activities.

It came down to a lack of understanding about what makes Marco who he was. His sensory and learning needs were creating much of his anxiety. The routines and structure decreased his anxiety because he knew what to expect, but when he had two different houses to go to with a lack of carry over and lack of consistency, Marco started to really struggle. He would have difficulties in each house, and it carried over into school and all his social activities. It was like Marco was a different child.

The blame for his change in behaviors was the separation. The parents blamed each other. People external to the family and the school also thought that was the difference. Yes, it partly was, but it may not have been the actual separation that was only affecting him. It was more the lack of consistency and routines that he craved daily. Each parent needed to understand what their subconscious priorities were doing to affect Marco.

When teachers and therapists have differing underlying priorities, the child's focus may be different when they are in that environment. Some classrooms I have worked in have excessive rules and structures that make it hard for children to follow. Other classrooms have no structure or order, as the focus is on having fun and keeping everyone happy. Balance is key for children. They need to feel that they belong and are significant, but understanding boundaries within a system helps guide children's actions and behaviors. Having fun is terrific, as long as it is respectful and appropriate to those around them. I have worked with children who have been the subject of jokes in a classroom, even from their teacher, to get a laugh from the class. Finding joy in other people's misery or playing practical jokes at the expense of others are not acceptable in any environment. It can be disheartening and very damaging for that student. I have also worked with teachers who are so supportive and enthusiastic for students' success that children try harder and achieve more because they believe they are capable. Children in each environment will respond differently.

Having lifestyle priorities can be advantageous for helping children. These priorities help create strong leaders, have structure and order, and teach us how to have fun and enjoy life. Recognizing your priorities, balancing them, and understanding how they can affect children and the choices we make as adults will influence how children learn to form their priorities. These examples also emphasize the importance of collaboration of those around the child to support a child effectively.

Competing External Priorities

It is not only our internal priorities that can impact a child. In our society, we have so many external competing priorities in our day, such as work, school, sports, clubs, committees, family, and friends, to name a few. The challenge is that each of these priorities competes for the limited time and attention that we have in our day. What we focus on, whether it is our choice or others choosing for us, can impact the rest of the priorities.

Tran worked at a large marketing firm in his town. He started there in an entry-level position. He had a degree in marketing, and his dream job was to be an account manager for some big marketing clients. Tran also was a father of three active and busy children. He worked hard at his job and was good at what he did, but he was told he needed to put in extra hours, take clients out for dinners, and travel more if he wanted to be considered for a promotion. Tran's three children were all competitive dancers. They loved to dance and were really good. The dance studio thought they had real potential to excel in competitions. Yet this would mean that they would have to practice at the studio five to six nights per week. One of his children also struggled at school with fine motor activities. He had difficulty printing, coloring, and doing up zippers and buttons, so the school suggested some therapy. Another one of his children struggled in reading, and their teacher thought it would be a good idea to get some extra reading help two days a week after school. Tran also had a partner who worked out of the home and was an emergency physician. This meant shift work for the partner and could mean long hours. Then they still had to fit in meal times, time for homework, friends, and family.

Sasha was a single mother of two children. She worked two jobs just to keep their home and pay the bills. Her children went to care before and after school, and when she picked them up, they would have some dinner before she would leave them with a grandparent so that she could go to her next job. Sasha's focus was on providing a home, food, and clothing for her and her children. She was doing her best to keep them afloat. The challenge was that this didn't leave Sasha much time to spend helping her children with homework or incorporating any therapy suggestions.

It may sound overwhelming to read, but this is the reality of our society today. Parents receive many suggestions, prompts, or recommendations for what they should do, and it can seem overwhelming. Whether right or wrong, our society is built on the idea that you need to be, do, and achieve more to be successful.

If one parent decides that work is the priority, often with a good intention of supporting the family and providing for them, it will mean less time spent at home. It may be their only option, and it can then impact the children. If a parent feels that children should be the priority, it could affect the family's income and create some additional stress. With less income, it can mean having less food, losing a home, or decreased ability to participate in extracurricular activities that a child wants.

Then add on if a parent is asked to be a part of a committee or a family member is ill, such as a child or grandparent, and requires extra care outside the home.

These competing and differing priorities will impact how much a parent or caregiver can take on in relation to a child.

James was Tran's child who struggled with holding a pencil and other fine motor activities. The therapist had many great ideas for James to work on at home to practice these skills. Yet, with Tran's competing priorities and lack of support from his partner, many recommendations never were done.

It all comes down to choices. A parent or caregiver needs to think about what choices they are making, what needs to be given a priority at any given moment. As someone working with the child, we cannot choose for a parent, but we need to be part of the conversation about what reality looks like for them. If a parent can only work with a child for five minutes before they go to bed or during a commute in a car, what would be your top recommendation for that child? If a teacher wants a parent to read with a child for 15 minutes each day, but a parent only has 5 minutes, what is a 5-minute activity? We need to change how we communicate based on the family's reality and understanding what competing priorities exist. There needs to be space to have those open conversations in a nonjudgmental way.

Maybe we need to change the way we look at helping a child. Should it be a separate activity, or should learning be integrated into daily activities? In the book *Learning How to Learn*,[17] Oakley et al. discuss memory-enhancing techniques to learn new information. One of the suggestions was to pair the method with something you already do, as this helps make those connections in the brain and strengthens learning.[17]

How can therapeutic goals and educational goals be integrated into a daily routine to become part of the everyday activities? How do we change the conversations to be more productive? How can we work together as a team?

In the next chapter, I will discuss the importance of a collaborative approach and what that looks like.

Generational Differences

Who lives at home with a child can also affect what happens in the house, especially if those people are involved in raising a child or participating in therapy goals. Some families live in a multigenerational home. It means that they have grandparents or great grandparents living with them. Some families may not live with grandparents, but have grandparents who are actively involved. When there are multiple generations involved in the child's care, it is vital to understand how this can affect a child. As I discussed at the beginning of the book, the era in which you were born can impact your mindset, opinions, and beliefs. Raising children then and now is very different. Understanding some of the differences can be important.

It was more common in the past that a parent would be home with children growing up. Now it is more common in a two-parent family to have both employed. Sometimes this is by choice, but the cost of living has dramatically changed in the last couple of generations, requiring two incomes to afford living expenses.

Technology has also changed the most in the last 30 years. It has changed the way we send and receive information. It has put access to information literally at our fingertip. Children no longer need to ask as many questions from parents or grandparents, as the answers can be found on their phones or tablets. If they are curious about anything, good or bad, they can search and have answers in minutes. It has changed how children socialize with others and has impacted how we move around, experience, and physically explore the world. Technology has many positives in helping those who have trouble communicating to have a voice. Still, on the negative, the effects of technology have tapped into our brain chemistry and make us more dependent and attached to our devices.

Just yesterday, I was having a conversation about technology with my children. They were frustrated that a movie was taking a long time to load. Mind you, it was only a matter of minutes. I reminded them that when streaming first started and the internet was slower, it would take hours to download movies or shows. Then, to go back even further, we had to drive to the video store to get a video to watch. There would only be one copy for some videos, and if it were out, you would have to wait till it was back in.

With this increase in information, we are also more aware of what is going on globally. News is instantly sent to our phones. We get alerts when something bad happens nearby. We can see personal footage from people's phones of incidents across the world. This awareness has also increased the fear for children's freedom to roam outside. In past generations, children used to wander more freely and return home when the street lights came on.

Additionally, our awareness of individual and racial diversity and equality has changed. The freedom to be, act, and share what makes you unique is expressed more than in past generations, especially, in the last years with the advent of Black Lives Matter, the Truth and Reconciliation Commission, #Metoo movement, and the global pandemic. Our understanding and interpretation of these movements will be impacted by your personal story.

With all of the changes that have occurred, it can make it especially hard for a child if both the parents and grandparents are involved with raising a child and they disagree on their approach. If the parents' expectations differ from those with a grandparent, the child may be unsure of how to act and behave. It can especially stand out if there is fighting or negative comments expressed, such as "I would never raise my child like this" or "My method worked; my children turned out fine." This judgment level can be making it hard as a parent to balance your own choices versus those of your parents.

There are benefits to having support from family members, as it can ease the strain on a parent or caregiver, especially when children are young. As the saying goes, it indeed does "take a village to raise a child." There is value in building relationships outside of the immediate family for a child, and creating the bond can help a child feel connection and love from grandparents. So that this is a beneficial relationship for everyone, parents need to have conversations with those involved in caring for a child. Communicating the needs of the child, especially when it comes to their sensory and learning needs, is crucial. It is valuable to understand each person's perspective and validate those feelings. Setting boundaries regarding the responsibilities of the child and having clear expectations set for how help is received will be an important starting point. Sometimes, grandparents can have a strong bond with a child, which can be a positive asset in helping the child's needs.

It is vital to understand when multigenerational families are involved in the care of the child. The differing perspectives can influence how a child feels and how they accept recommendations. It is especially important to understand if the grandparent has full custody of a child.

When Support Is Not Available

For some people, access to family support is not an option. Whether it be physical distance or choice, it can feel a bit more challenging to do it alone, especially when a parent is trying to manage a job, the household, and provide care for their child. It can be stressful and lonely for a parent, especially if a child has additional needs.

Going back to the beginning of this chapter, those working with the child need to be aware of competing priorities within a caregiver's life. Whether or not there is additional support, the conversation needs to be open to understand what is within the caregiver's current capacity to support the child. If someone is struggling, it will be necessary to work with them to find the support they need to take care of them.

When parents or caregivers themselves are not willing or able to actively participate with their child, ensuring the child's safety is the number one focus. It is more than a choice. It is a legal responsibility. If the child is safe, including the parent in conversations is still valuable, as it exposes them to knowledge and makes them feel that sense of belonging that we all desire.

Starting the Conversation for Support

To begin, it is essential to remind caregivers that support doesn't only come in the form of relatives. Within a community, there are often resources and assistance available. Sometimes, it is a matter of not knowing that they exist or how to connect with them.

To help a child function to their capacity, it may be necessary to provide resources to the parent. Like the mom at the beginning of this chapter who was struggling with depression, the recommendation we had for the child will not be useful until the mom has resources to help her, or other supports are available for the children. Likewise, the child at the beginning of the book who came to school hungry and exhausted, the support needs to begin with the parent to meet the child's basic needs.

It goes back to understanding the current situation and capacity and setting the priorities. It requires the openness and vulnerability of all the parties involved to acknowledge that they need help. People may be willing to help, but they don't know how they can help unless they know what is going on.

The first goal is to outline what help you need. The more specific you can be, the more people can step in.

The next step is to know who it is you are talking to. See if it is within their capacity to be able to support the current situation. What is going on in their life at the moment? Reaching out to another mom struggling with her children may not be your best resource.

The last step is to create a collaborative plan or approach to helping the child or family. Assisting a child requires understanding the child's needs and consistency in how those needs are managed. It involves parents and caregivers having similar objectives and goals and clear and straightforward communication. Learning about setting boundaries and expectations in the home environment can lead to the structure a child needs.

When working with children, family support can be vital in helping a child to reach their potential. Yet as we have seen through this chapter, it may not be as straightforward as expecting every parent to be able to give their full support and commitment. We can't change the way the world works, just like we can't change how a child's brain reacts to the world. What we can do is create a space that gives knowledge to those involved in raising a child. I believe that knowledge is power, and it helps us to make better informed choices and decisions that can support a child.

Chapter Reflections

1. How can parents' differing backgrounds impact a child?
2. What are lifestyle priorities?
3. Why can external priorities compete with a child's needs?
4. How can generational differences impact a child's upbringing?
5. How can a family find external support?

11 Collaborative Problem Solving

So, what do we do now? We have reached the point where we have looked at many different aspects that make up a child. The information provides us with a clearer picture of who this child is and how they function in the world. What do we do with this information, and how does it help us from this point on?

For those brought up in North America, Thanksgiving dinner is often a big celebration. For those not familiar with Thanksgiving, think of it as any family holiday meal. You may be wondering how we jumped to Thanksgiving dinner, but stick with me for a moment. Thanksgiving often brings people together with a vision to celebrate a meal together and spend time together in one house. All the people who come for dinner contribute something to the meal. Depending on their skills or specialties, they bring their creations. One family brings the cranberry ring, one family brings the green bean casserole, one family brings the wine, one family brings the stuffing, and the host makes the turkey. Each person's contribution to the dinner is important, and the dinner wouldn't be complete without it. To reach the vision of sitting down to the meal together at the same time, some planning needs to go into place so that each person's dish will be ready at the same time. Some items take longer to make, and others take no time at all. It involves working together to share the space and understand the plan.

If something were to go wrong in this space, as it did one year for us, you learn how to pivot and make some changes to still get to your vision. One year, right in the middle of the dinner preparations, a glass shattered into a million pieces, ending up in the majority of the prepared food. It meant that almost all the food needed to be thrown out, as you couldn't see the glass pieces. We had to quickly work together to develop a new plan to reach the goal of celebrating a meal together. It may not have been the meal we had planned, but we were still working towards the same vision and goal.

What does this have to do with what we have learned this far about the story of a child? Coming together with all the information we have learned and developing a plan for the child is like bringing a family together for Thanksgiving dinner. Some key people are invited to the table—each person with their role, experience, and knowledge. Each person brings equal value to the table. The actions are all focused on the outcome. What if someone couldn't make

DOI: 10.4324/9781003166405-11

the dinner? For those who couldn't make the dinner, their input is still important and valuable. What is also important is all the information that they didn't hear from those who did make it.

So, let's talk about who is invited to the table. In the world of business, these are known as the key players or the system partners. Who is it important to communicate and discuss this information with?

Key Players

The key players or system partners are those people who have a vested interest or responsibility for what the story is about. If the story is about a child, then the child would be a key person. If the child is capable in any way, they should be a part of the conversation and included in discussions and planning. If the child cannot participate yet, the caregiver becomes the key person, but as the child continues to develop, this may change, and they can be brought into the conversation.

This is so important because when people are making plans for you, you want to make sure they align with what your goals are. Think about if someone told you that you would be a pilot growing up, and you didn't have a choice. The problem is you are scared of heights and get motion sickness every time you fly. The choice that someone else made for you may not match your needs or desires, of which both are necessary for an activity to be successful.

The parents or caregivers are sources for another key player. As we discussed in the last chapter, they may or may not have the capacity to help a child at this moment, but they are legally responsible for making decisions and need to be a part of the conversation. This could include grandparents, parents, or guardians.

All of the rest of the people invited to "Thanksgiving dinner" will be anyone else who directly influences the child. At school, this would include any teacher who teaches that child, teacher's assistants, child and youth workers, the principal, and vice-principal.

Outside of school, the key players are people who are involved in supporting the child in some way. It includes your family doctor, specialists, therapists, psychologists, social workers, and even coaches or club leaders. Sometimes, it is harder to get those outside of the school together in the same room for the conversation, but their information is valuable, as what they may have noticed about a child can affect a child in other areas.

Why is it important to know who the key players/system partners are?

Each person mentioned earlier at some point will have direct influence or responsibility of the child. When that person is in charge of a child, they can better support the child if they have information that may influence their choices.

Craig was part of a kids' club. He loved to participate in the activities and be a part of the group. He was adventurous and creative. Craig also struggled with anxiety and was hypersensitive to noises, which could make it difficult for him to follow instructions, and occasionally he would get lost on what he was doing. At this point, his anxiety would increase, and he would tend to get upset. If Craig went to the kids' club and his leader didn't know what bothered Craig, it would be hard for that leader to know what approach would help him. In this case, the information is key. Craig's leader may not need to know Craig's entire history, but understanding his noise sensitivity and how to best help him through it would make Craig's and his group's experience so much better. Craig's leader could ask Craig what the best approach would be to help Craig stay on task. If Craig's leader were to discover an activity that engaged Craig and helped him work through some of his anxiety, that information may help others who work with Craig and is worth being shared.

If we look at all the people we have mentioned so far in this chapter, who is responsible for creating an environment that can help children reach their greatest potential?

EVERYONE.

I want to say that again. EVERYONE. Anyone who is tasked with engaging with a child needs to be working towards the same goal for that child. It is the collaboration of people that will have the greatest impact on the success of the child.

What Does Collaboration Mean?

Collaboration means working together to come up with a plan. It means that everyone is part of the plan, including the child if possible. Going back to the Thanksgiving dinner, collaboration means that everyone brought something to the dinner to make the dinner complete.

When you collaborate, it involves discussing and negotiating to come up with a solution. It requires problem solving a plan and how to work towards that plan.

What is key about collaborating is that you may not always agree on the ideas presented. Each person brings their views, backgrounds, and experiences. Collaborating means that you come together as equals to discuss the different perspectives and develop the best options for the child. Someone else in the group may have thought of an idea that others hadn't considered, and we want to make sure that we give everyone a chance to participate. To keep everyone on track and focused, creating a plan helps to ensure that all the ideas are aligned in the same direction.

Making a "Business Plan" to Guide You

When we think about a business plan, we often think about big businesses like Nike or Apple. We don't often think about a family as a mini business. Yet it is. I don't call myself this often, but I am the Chief Mom Officer. I oversee the day-to-day ongoing of the business. We have to meet short-term and long-term goals, and I have people who are dependent on this business to run effectively for their well-being, and on top of that, we need to maintain a budget. If we only functioned day to day, our business would be in a bit of ongoing chaos. We could have financial unrest if we didn't watch our budget, and we could have some interoffice disputes, otherwise known as sibling rivalry. Some people don't have a desire to own a business or worry about running a business. They enjoy working in an already organized structure, as it provides the boundaries and instills that sense of belonging and security. Yet a family needs to run like a business in order to thrive and not just survive. The feeling of being a part of an organization or group is similar to what children desire when they are part of the family. As much as we may not want to lead an organization, being part of a group like a family involves many of the same benefits and challenges as running a business.

What makes any business more effective and efficient is if everyone is on the same page: meaning, everyone is working towards the same vision with the same mission. Most business plans don't look to the past. They often use the past as a reference, but spend their time looking to the future. It helps to guide where we are headed. So far, a child's view in this book has been looking at where they are now and where they have come from. All that has shaped a child to this point has shown us how their story is developing. Looking past this point into the future is where we need to come up with a plan.

As parents, we often have dreams for our children. These dreams involve them growing up to be happy, independent, and successful adults. Sometimes in the thick of childhood, we forget that these children will grow up to be adults. We need to help them express the vision of where they want to be, or if communication is challenging, start them on a path towards where we see them growing up to be.

Like I discussed about my family business, there are two ways to run a business. One way is to take each day as it comes and see what happens, leading to potential chaos. The second way is to set a goal and spend each day reaching towards that goal. The first way could mean aimlessly wandering with no guidance or direction. The second way has focus and clarity to a specific purpose.

Imagine your child wants to be an NBA basketball player. That is their dream. Whether or not it becomes a reality is not the question, but what you do to help them get to their vision is going to be the key. If you never teach a child how to play basketball, they will not be getting closer to their dream. Yet, if instead, you look for every opportunity to expose them to basketball, their goals may get closer to reality. It is how you align your actions with your dreams.

Now, if you take that dream and share it with others, those you share it with may now be invested in helping you find opportunities for your child to get closer to their dream as well. You are then collaborating on a dream.

Setting up a dream for your child is like creating a vision for where you see them in the future. It is about looking at the end game. When you have a vision for your child, it looks beyond today and tomorrow and gives us a destination to strive for. There's a quote that states *"You will only hit what you aim at."*

When you have that vision, all the decisions you make need to align with that vision, and all the goals you set need to bring you a step closer to the end goal.

It's just like running a business and having employees working for you. They need to know the company's vision to align their jobs to match that vision. When everyone is on the same page, the team's collaboration will increase the success of reaching the goals. The vision for Thanksgiving dinner was to sit down for a nice meal and have some great social time together. Each person made that possible because they all knew what the vision was and contributed to it by bringing their part of the meal.

What does this look like for a child, and why is this important?

Vision

When children are young, adults often ask them what they want to be when they grow up. This can change a thousand times, but eventually, as they experience and explore the world, they start to gravitate towards specific ideas. This becomes a child's vision for their future. It is the goal that they want to reach. Sometimes, this can be skewed by those around them, such as pressures, fears, or disappointments, but the vision should be aligned in the child's best interest. The child should not be a pilot if they are afraid of flying, nor should a child have a goal of being a doctor if they are scared of blood.

Depending on the child's capacity, the vision can be created in conjunction with the child or started by the team around them. If a child can't understand or decide what they want to be, parents, caregivers, and key players can also create an idea of a vision for them to start them in a direction. It may be less specific, but it involves creating a future idea the child could reach. I've heard it said that a vision is just a dream with a dose of reality. The vision should have nothing to do with a label a child's been given or a disability. We should never make our vision of a child limit their potential. Think about Nic Vujicic[8] who we discussed earlier in the book, born with no arms and legs. At the beginning of his life, there were few expectations of what he would accomplish. Yet he far exceeded what they thought he would be capable of. When we think of a child's potential, we should start with an idea of what we believe is achievable and then go beyond that in our vision to something that exceeds that.

In my early days as an occupational therapist, I had a passion for finding ways to modify sports equipment to increase inclusivity in sports. One of my early clients was a gentleman with quadriplegia. He had very little use of his arms and no use of his legs, but his dream was to sail a sailboat independently. If you have a dream and it becomes your vision, it can manifest into reality because you start to focus on clues and cues that align with that vision. He was able to find a sailing club that had a weighted keel sailboat, which means it had less chance of flipping over. He researched other people with quadriplegia who had tried, and he hired a sailing coach to help him. The one challenge he had was that he had difficulty staying in the boat's seat with his decreased trunk stability. I helped him create a more stable harness that would harness him into the seat. He needed to get out of the chair quickly, so I needed to research ways that he could release his harness quickly in case of emergency. It just so happened that after he asked me to help him with his harness, I was on an airplane and realized that the airplane buckles were designed so that it made it relatively easy for anyone to get out of the buckle. I reached out to the airplane seat belt company and created a release system using airplane buckles. He was able to use this harness and the weighted boat to sail independently.

In this case, the gentleman created the vision and then reached out to all the different system partners to help him reach his idea and meet all the goals necessary. His dream became a reality.

Have you ever thought about where you want to be in 10 years or 20 years? What is your vision, and how are you working towards that vision?

The impact of a vision is that it gives alignment to everything else that goes on in a child's life. Like the basketball player at the beginning of this chapter, the choices you make need to align with that goal. If a vision for a child is to be able to live independently as an adult, then everything leading up to that goal needs to work towards independence.

The key is that when you come up with a vision for a child, you need to share this with those key people we discussed earlier. Just like a business, you have system partners that are a part of or invested in the business. In a child's life, these key people are the people involved in helping a child achieve their goals, and sharing the vision creates that clarity and focus that's going to align all the rest of the plans and activities in the same path.

Steven struggled with communication and focus. He was behind in school and required a lot of one-on-one assistance. The parents' vision for Steven was for him to be able to live independently in the community. They shared this vision with all the people around Steven. This included the school, health care professionals, family members, and community support. Every decision made was checked for alignment with the vision to find out how it helped create his independence. As Steven was falling farther and farther behind in school, at one of the school meetings, it was suggested that Steven have someone scribe for him during class. The idea of having someone scribe for Steven meant that someone was going to do the work that he needed to do for writing. The question was asked: "How does this align with the vision for Steven?" It didn't. It made it more convenient at the moment, but in no way did it help Steven become more independent. Because there was a vision that they could align the goals with, the question was asked: "What other options are there?" At this point, the suggestion came out that Steven could learn to use talk to text. In this example, teaching Steven how to use this type of technology would increase his independence and decrease his reliance on others. It was more aligned with the vision for Steven.

Just like Steven and his independence or the gentleman learning to sail, these visions need to have some paths to get them there. I have always loved this quote: "Goals are visions and dreams with work clothes on."[26]

Creating Goals

The goals become the specifics for how we can reach a vision. Looking at Steven's example, the vision is for him to live independently in the community. The goals within that vision would be that he would be able to understand money, communicate his needs, cook for himself, clean for himself, and have a job. Having goals clarifies what we need to do to help us get to his end goal.

Businesses often have short-term goals and long-term goals. The difference with these goals is the length of time it would take to achieve them. It may take longer to teach Steven how to cook a meal, which is a long-term goal, but he may learn how to chop vegetables as a short-term goal. If one of Steven's goals is to cook for himself, a short-term goal would be to learn meal planning and grocery shopping. Those would be considered short-term goals within the long-term goal. If another goal is to understand money, a short-term goal would be to do simple addition and subtraction. It would not be necessary to struggle through complex algebra, as that is not required to understand money.

With a younger child, if a goal is for a child to dress independently, the short-term goal is when they can successfully achieve part of that goal. For instance, can they put their socks on, or can they put their underwear on? Each short-term goal lets us re-evaluate and check in to ensure that we're moving in the right direction.

This is what we do as occupational therapists. The vision and goals of what we are trying to achieve is the occupation discussed at the beginning of the book. It is the activity that a person is trying to do. By separating it into smaller, more manageable pieces, we can increase someone's ability to succeed at the task they are trying to do. From the learning needs discussed in Chapter 6, we know that creating building blocks in the brain helps build successful learning pathways. Creating goals helps to make those building blocks.

We have determined that goals are valuable for working towards a vision. Goals need to have some boundaries to ensure that they are reasonable and appropriate for what we need. In business, you often hear of goal setting as related to SMART goals. It is the same for life goals. Smart goals are goals that are specific, measurable, achievable, relevant, and timely. If you have a goal for one day doing a 5 K run, it may never happen, as you haven't set a specific plan or a timeline for achieving the goal. If you instead say that you will do a 5 K run in May of next year in the town close to you, you now have the specifics for your goal, making it more likely that you will achieve it. Within that larger goal, you can now set smaller goals that are also measurable: such as each month, you will add on half a km to your current distance for training.

The same specific types of goals should be used when working with children. It gives those working with the child the ability to have timelines with check-ins to see how the goals are progressing. By setting goals for children at school, we know what the focus will be for some time, and we can check in to see if that goal was achieved and advance them as needed.

Mission Statement

With having a vision and goals, I believe that it is essential, just like other companies, to have a statement that sets the framework behind your vision. We often hear about companies' mission statements, and it is why they exist. Google's mission statement is "to organize the world's information and make it universally accessible and useful."[27] In comparison, Nike's mission is "To bring inspiration and innovation to every athlete* in the world. *If you have a body, you are an athlete."[28] A mission statement is short and straightforward, but it focuses on what you want to achieve. It is the boundaries behind your vision.

In his book *The 7 Habits of Highly Effective People*, Stephen Covey[29] emphasized that having a mission statement for your own life and your family is like having a set of guiding principles like the constitution. Our mission statement comes from what we collectively believe and what the family has as a foundation. Stephen Covey's strong belief in having a mission statement aligns with the ideas of using this mission statement to give meaning and purpose to all the decisions we make daily.[29]

In my family, we have developed a mission statement that integrates our core values. Each child was able to add one idea that was incorporated into our mission statement. In my family, our mission is to love unconditionally, choose kindness, help when help is needed, seek out adventures, and enjoy the process. In creating this mission statement, when we make choices or something happens, we can go back and compare it to our family mission. For example, if children are upset and fighting, at that moment, we can ask them if they are showing love or choosing kindness to one another.

In creating Steven's vision of independence, a mission statement could be for Steven to thrive in an inclusive environment where he is happy, feels loved and understood, and celebrates his uniqueness. Creating independence for Steven is only a good vision if it keeps aligned with him thriving, being happy, and feeling loved. If creating his independence causes seclusion and feeling unloved, we did not match the vision to his mission.

Having a mission statement like this ensures that all those involved focus on helping Steven make sure that he is thriving. It is valuable to think about your mission statement, about what you would live by, and the guiding principles that help you decide what decision is right for you.

Do you have a personal or family mission statement?

Creating Collaboration and Family Meetings

When you create a vision, goals, and a mission statement, you create an alignment of purpose. It is like a guide for the path you want to take. The way may not always go in a straight line, but it keeps us moving forward. When you collaborate, as we discussed earlier, it means working together, and if you have a framework to work under, it keeps the focus and clarifies what the plan is. When working with a team of people, decisions then go through the framework's filter and require less contemplating. It is vital to set up regular check-in points with those involved to ensure things are on track.

The same should be done in a family. If you have a family mission statement, vision, and goals, you can create meetings with the family to discuss any family decisions. Teaching children how to make decisions based on beliefs and values helps them understand and learn how to make good choices. Including children in this process also makes them feel that they have a sense of belonging and are valued family members.

Without this, every decision may just be based on getting through one problem at a time. Just like the suggestion to get a scribe to help Steven write, it would help at the moment, but would not help him long term.

Collaboration involves anyone who is a part of the group. When working with a child, this can include many people who are part of the team. No matter their job or their skills, whatever they are doing to work with the child needs to be working towards that common goal. That means that anytime somebody new is introduced to the child, they should learn the child's story and learn about the vision, mission, and set of goals. In a family, every family member is part of the group as well and should be included in the discussions.

How we communicate will be different depending on the group of people. The school setting is much more involved with a child, as the child will spend most of their time there outside of being at home. When dealing with health care professionals, we often don't have that same amount of time, but it is still essential for them to understand the child's whole story.

How to communicate with each group and work effectively together as a team will be discussed in the next two chapters.

Chapter Reflections

1. What does Thanksgiving dinner have to do with collaborative problem solving?
2. Who is responsible for creating an environment that can help children reach their potential?
3. Why is it important to have a vision for a child?
4. How can you align goals to the child's vision?
5. Why is it important for families to create a mission statement?

12 Communication With the School

Children spend the majority of their waking time during the week at school and dedicated to school or school-related activities. This includes getting ready for school, dropping off, picking up, and any school work that is sent home. That is why the people involved with the child at school play a significant role in a child's life. Communication between parents and school is key to helping children at school and carrying over what is learned at school to home and vice versa. Helping children thrive is about consistency and collaboration. Including the school input into creating the vision and goals for a child can help create some of the collaboration needed to help a child succeed.

Rayna was very quiet and often disengaged in class. It meant that she would be in class, but rarely participate. She would complete all her homework, but would often ask to go home, as she would say that she wasn't feeling well. Rayna didn't engage with many students at recess or lunch and mainly stayed to herself. Rayna's parents noticed that she did not like to go to school and often resisted and would again say she wasn't feeling well. She seemed okay at home, but didn't like when she had to go to any activities outside of the house, including watching her sister play volleyball or go to anyone else's home for dinner. As Rayna was a calm child both at home and at school, her parents and the school didn't even notice that her behavior was an issue. They didn't realize that Rayna was spending most of her day feeling overwhelmed by the environment. The overwhelm was activating her primitive brain, but instead of going into the fight response, she was going into the flight response and withdrawing from all activities. In Rayna's class, several other students also had significant struggles in the classroom. One would get loud and often yell at the teacher, or push his desk, or throw his books on the floor when he didn't want to do something. Another student would cry a lot if he were ever called on or frustrated with an activity. Within the same classroom, another student would self-regulate by humming to herself and tapping her hands.

This can be a common picture of a classroom experience. There is a class full of students with a varying degree of needs in one space. There is only one teacher and maybe an EA for a small period of time. The teacher is focused on teaching the lessons and moving ahead with the lesson plans. It is often the students who disrupt the teacher that become the focus, or the teacher tries to

DOI: 10.4324/9781003166405-12

ignore the behaviors and speaks over them. The disruptions get more intense till the teacher and student are at odds and may result in the student being sent out of the class.

In all that is happening in the classroom, a student like Rayna is often overlooked. Not intentionally, as she can get her work done, and she doesn't disrupt the class. Yet, she is struggling in the class and not being noticed. How can someone like Rayna get seen? How does someone like Rayna get support at the school for her needs?

This is where Rayna's parents need to get involved. Although they may not understand what is going on with Rayna, they need to start communication with the school to understand Rayna better. Creating a good teacher–parent relationship is essential for the success of a child at school. It can be challenging for teachers to have the time and energy to meet every child's needs in the classroom and stay in touch with every family. Yet, we know that the collaboration between both sides can make the job easier at home and school. Effective communication is one of the most important parts of the relationship between school and those around the child.

A teacher can gain significant insight into a student's life because they get to see them in a variety of settings throughout the day. This includes them interacting with adults, peers, sitting in class, break times, and gym class. They also can see how the child processes information through their academic expectations. A teacher's role in a child's story is significant, and educators need to understand the impact they can have on how the story unfolds throughout the year. Sometimes, we rely on the knowledge of a therapist to help understand a child. This is also valuable, but a therapist's experience will be different from that of a teacher. I will detail this in the next chapter, but a therapist works with a child for a very short time, potentially half an hour at a time. It can be once or twice a week, but more commonly once every two or three weeks. What a teacher has the capacity to see and do on a regular basis will have more impact on a child than what a therapist can do in half an hour. This is why a teacher's role is so significant, and the collaboration between the therapist and the teacher can have a more substantial impact on a child.

The question comes up repeatedly: "Whose responsibility is it to help children reach their potential?" The answer is EVERYONE. So, figuring out a way to tap into all the children in the classroom will make the whole class succeed.

Is this easy? Of course not.
Is it important? 100%.
Can it take some time to get to know everyone? Certainly.
Will it make it more efficient in the end? 100%.

What if I gave you a task to serve a meal to 100 people this evening, and then I told you that you had five hours to prepare the space and cook the meal? I tasked 20 people to help you make this meal. With the time restraints, you have to be very efficient in getting the tasks done. What is the first thing you would do? Would you tell everyone to pick something and get started, or would you find out what everyone is capable of and put them on tasks that match their abilities?

I think that for efficiency, you would choose the latter. If you spend the time at the beginning to understand who has cooked before, washed and cut vegetables, baked before, set tables before, and cleaned before, you could organize your workforce into an efficient group. The time you spend speaking with each person and allowing them to share their strengths or weaknesses would not only make it run smoothly, but you have also now recognized and validated their contribution to the task at hand.

Using the language we learned in the last chapter to describe this scenario, you had a vision for what needs to get done, and you have created goals for each group of students to focus on. This creates alignment and focus and keeps everyone on task. To ensure that people treat each other well, you could include a mission or values statement for your group, including treating each other with respect, being kind to one another, and having fun. It sets the guidelines for the activity and how everyone should work together.

So why don't we often think about classrooms like this? Sometimes, I have heard from teachers that there isn't time to spend getting to know each student and understand their needs, or that it is the role of other people within the school to figure out a student's needs. Dr. Ross Greene's definition of good teaching "means being responsive to the hand you've been dealt" (p. 182).[19] It means being fully aware of what the children in the class need and how a teacher can best support them.

Throughout this book, I have shared many different stories about children in school settings. Children who thrive in the school environment and children who struggle. So, what is it that makes that difference?

I believe it is the connection within the classroom. It is the connection between the teacher and the other students. It is the sense of belonging, love, and safety that is necessary for our being. If children feel that they belong, they can be authentically themselves, and they are supported for their needs. This is often when we see children soar. I have watched this with children I work with and with my own children, how each year can make a big difference depending on who is leading the class. It is the same with who leads an organization. The feeling you have as part of the group can make a big difference to a person's sense of belonging. Creating that sense of community amongst your students makes everyone a valued participant, and we learn to help and recognize each other's needs.

So, how do we connect all the pieces? Throughout this book, we have learned a lot of information that helps form a child's story. Sharing this information in the right way will affect how the child is portrayed and accepted. Even within the school environment, there can be multiple people involved in the well-being of the child. How we communicate about a child can define the relationship and how the child feels supported. It is essential to allow each person to share the part of the child's story that they have experienced and listen to the others to understand how to build an effective relationship.

School-to-Parent Relationships

The school-to-parent relationship needs to be a two-way communication. It should be open in both directions with the person directly in charge of the student, often the classroom teacher. What is happening with a child at home can impact what is happening with the same child at school and vice versa. If a parent is ill or a relative passed away, it can affect a child's emotions at school during that time. Likewise, if a child was injured at school or did something inappropriate and was disciplined, it may affect a child's behavior when they get off the bus. I recently worked with a parent who told me that the best years her son has had at school were when the teacher's communication was the most open. This teacher would send a message to the parent to let the mom know when she would be away for a day. This gave the mom the ability to prepare her son for a change in routine. The mom would likewise send a message to the teacher when something happened in the morning, and the teacher might not push the child as much during the day. With this communication, there were less outbursts in the class, and it made the environment better for everyone, including the child.

Behaviors that happen at school in the classroom may also be a sign of something that is bothering them or they are struggling with at school, but this may not be something that a child struggles with at home. A teacher needs to discuss this with parents or caregivers, as it can help to gain an understanding of what may be causing the challenges. It could be a variety of things we have already covered, including the physical environment, the people, or the work.

In the same way, behaviors that happen at home may not happen at school, but can be related. It is also essential to understand and communicate these findings, as it can affect what happens at home. One of my children would get off the bus, throw his bag on the ground, and have a meltdown at that moment. He would be in this state for nearly an hour after school every day. The teacher said that everything was fine with him at school. He played well with friends and was quiet in class. Yet, I believe it took all of his energy to keep that up at school, and he was utterly depleted when he got home and was still experiencing the tension from school.

I began to learn that he could not focus in class due to the sounds in the classroom, and he was often lost and trying to figure out what to do. An example in one art class was that he had to draw a red bird sitting on a stick with leaves on it. He drew a bird, but it was blue and was sitting on a stick with no leaves. Although maybe biased by his mother's opinion, his drawing was amazing, but he was marked poorly on his drawing because he only followed half the instructions. The teacher never realized what was going on with him in class, because it never stood out to her. He was behind in all his subjects, but the response was that he was at least better than some of the other children in the class. The struggles that my son began to have in school that year escalated into a lot of negative self-talk at home, rage against his siblings, and resistance to go to school or do homework. Although a teacher may not see this at school, they need to recognize that some of the day's activities may be negatively impacting a child at home.

Within any school, teachers have a lot they must accomplish within a given year. It is not an easy job to keep everyone focused on moving ahead in the curriculum and ensuring everyone is safe throughout the day. Sometimes, so much focus may be on the tasks that need to get done, that it's hard to see why a child might be resisting, avoiding, or withdrawing from participating. When the focus changes to the behavior that a child exhibits instead of the reason, there is a misalignment between the child and the teacher. According to the teacher, my son was fine because he didn't act out, but another child in the class got angry and talked back when he was frustrated, so he was assessed as struggling more than my son. Anyone working with a child needs to maintain a curious mind and remember the complex stories of each child and how different children can express their struggles in different ways.

To build the school-to-parent relationship, it is valuable to start the conversation with those involved with the child, like the teacher, at the beginning of the school year. It should not be with just a transition team for a child; this should include the actual people who will be present with the child daily. Often, teachers will meet parents by the end of the first month of school, but often new transitions for children are the most difficult. Having this approach needs the open-mindedness of everyone involved. That way, the year can start positively, and the teacher is aware of some of the child's background. Building this connection is intended to be mutually beneficial. This means that by sharing this information, we hope parents can help teachers at school, and in return, it will help at home. Communicating the child's vision is important as is having them understand the story of who the child is, including the information learned through this book. It should be less about their diagnosis or disability and more about their capabilities, strengths, and what they are striving for.

If a child is receiving or in need of extra help at school, a child will be assessed or monitored to see if they require the help. At this point, strategies should be implemented on a trial basis to see if they are helping a child. If the child requires help consistently, a document referred to as an individualized education plan, or IEP, can be made to help meet that child's needs. It is a plan created for students who are having difficulty keeping up with the current curriculum or functioning in school. It is a legally binding document that sets in place the child's needs for the upcoming year. The IEP is intended to be a written document between the school, child, and parent. Once created, the school is required to uphold all that is written in it. The idea behind setting up an individualized plan ensures that the school will provide resources and accommodations for all academic, therapy, and physical learning opportunities and environments.

We want to ensure that all the goals and supports listed on the IEP are aligned with the child's overall vision and are appropriate for the child's needs. It is intended to be specific so that it can be evaluated to ensure that the goals of the IEP are met. It isn't easy to always know and understand what a child might need as the year progresses. Therefore, if a child is not doing well during the year, a meeting can be held to revise the IEP mid-year.

One concern I have about an IEP is that it is often focused on the problems that existed in the past. What it doesn't always account for is creating a plan for encouraging a child to learn new skills to fully reach their potential. For example, if a child struggled with doing their testing within the time allowed, an accommodation could be that they are allowed extra time for all their tests. What is not usually included is teaching the child new ways to study, decrease testing anxiety, or efficiently write a test. It is focused more on the problem that a child faces rather than understanding how to help a child find a solution. For example, a scribe is more often an option on an IEP for a child who has difficulty writing to solve the problem of slow output, rather than teaching a child how to print or write.

Another example may include a modification to the curriculum so that the child has less work, even though it may not be the work, but rather the eye–hand coordination to complete the work. By understanding more about who the child is, the goal is to create a document that works to the student's strengths and doesn't impede or prevent them from reaching their vision. An IEP should be a way for a child to function to their capacity in an environment that is not always accommodating. We need to remember when working with children that decisions made early in their life can change the trajectory of their future. We don't want the IEP to impede their future choices or goals. We need to be careful that the plan we set out for a child is not for the school's convenience or the adults, but is in the child's best interest.

The IEP is the underlying document for a child, which is intended to help a child throughout the year. Yet, sometimes, we can get caught up in the daily challenges that occur and look at the quickest and easiest way to solve those problems. I was once shown a video on YouTube, and I was asked to watch and count how many times the ball was passed back and forth. Because I was focused on counting the passing ball, I missed the fact that a gorilla walked through the scene. When the video was over, and the audience was asked how many saw the gorilla, very few raised their hand. Sometimes, when you're so focused on your task, you can often miss some of the other important information that is going on in the background.

When the focus becomes so much on a specific issue, it can spiral into something that does not help either the child or the school. I met with a mom recently who was telling me about her child and how his behavior had become the focus of all of his days at school. Because of his behavior, his time at school was shortened. Eventually, he was only allowed to come to school for one hour so that they could work on him behaving in that environment. The challenge was that to be prepared and for the staff to be safe, they would put on special safety equipment so that they would not get injured if something happened. It included wearing gloves, a padded vest, and sometimes a face shield. Think for a moment how that would make you feel as a child if the person you are trying to connect with is geared up with equipment that makes you feel as though something is significantly wrong with you. When I heard this, it reminded me of a jail guard. The focus was trying to control the results and change the outcome without changing the cause or understanding the trigger. Remember *a child will behave if they can*, so if the environment is set up with triggers that already escalate the primitive response to fight or flight, you will not see a behavior change.

What if we took that same child and, instead of focusing on academics or rule following, just allowed them to do activities that get them into that "just right" state? This approach would enable the caregiver to begin to build that bond or connection with the child. When a child feels safe and connected, they begin to build trust. This then allows us to slowly integrate some other activities into their day.

This is why it's important that whoever's working with a child understands the child's story. This child who was only allowed to come for one hour a day not only had significant sensory issues, but his mom was also going through some medical treatments for cancer at the time. Children have difficulty processing when something is happening to their parents, especially if their parent bonds are strong. He may not be able to express this unrest, but it makes it even more important for the effort to be made to make him feel safe and connected in the school environment.

Instead, let's look at the bigger picture, including those areas that I have discussed in this book so far, to understand some of the "why" behind the challenges. It can help us develop a solution that is focused on the vision and is proactive.

Understanding the School Environment

The school environment is a complex environment. As discussed in an earlier chapter, it has the physical elements of the school building, classrooms, and furniture, but also a unique social element, with a classroom of 10–30 children in one space, with often hundreds of students in the building. To maintain the organization and order within the school, there are often strict institutional elements affecting policies and procedures to keep children safe. These can be created within the school district or even from a government or labor policy. One of the policies is about behavior and is often a zero-tolerance policy. This policy intends to ensure that the safety of both staff and students is maintained at all times. The challenge is that, often, it is not the behavior that is the issue; it is whatever is triggering the behavior that needs the focus. In Dr. Greene's book *The Explosive Child*,[22] he writes that "years of research is crystal clear on two points: zero tolerance policies have made things worse, not better; and standard school disciplinary practices generally aren't effective for the students to who they are most frequently applied" (p. 228). Recall the idea that a child would control their behavior if they could, so disciplining someone without understanding what got them to that point will not necessarily change the future outcomes.

With 30 children and their watching eyes in the classroom, how a behavior is dealt with can be used to set an example to others as to what will be tolerated at this school. In some ways, using that method instills fear in the other children about what may happen if they do something similar. This should not be the intention of the choice of discipline. If you take anything away from this book, it should be that each person has their own story and deserves to be heard and understood. It is not to make an excuse, but instead a guide for the most effective way to help a child change their outward expression of an internal struggle.

Think about the boy who was only allowed to come to school for an hour at a time. He struggled with so many challenges at home with his mom, he was coming to school with his engine already revving at high, and anything would push him to his limit. The overwhelm of the sensory experience in the classroom, combined with his inability to hear and follow instructions, made him act out. Using his behavior and the response to it as a demonstration to others of what would be tolerated did not consider all of the other things he was experiencing.

So how do you navigate the world of policies and procedures? First, we can agree that they are set in place for the health and safety of those involved in an organization.

The key would be to try to identify the smaller signs of a child being stressed that precede any significant behavioral outburst. It is important to take the time to see these signs and understand what is affecting the child. Then you support them, create the appropriate outlets for the stress, and then work with them to learn how to self-regulate. This type of approach needs to be encouraged by the school's leadership, the board, and the governing organizations.

When there is a collective belief that children would do well if they could and that we should react not to the outward displays, but with a more profound curiosity about why this behavior is happening, we will begin to see a dramatic change. In a school board near me, the mission statement reads: "We educate and nurture hope in all learners to realize their full potential to transform the world." If we focus on this mission, we can ask ourselves: "Are we doing all we can to nurture hope in ALL learners," or "Are we helping ALL learners realize their full potential?"

It brings us back to creating that positive parent–school relationship and creating a supportive network of people around the child to help them navigate this ever-changing world. This can include the children within the classroom. Each child deserves to feel that they are part of a group. It should not be just the children who act out or require extra help that should get the attention. If you create an environment where children are encouraged to look out for one another and care for each other, regardless of their differences, it makes this an inclusive environment.

Just like my mother-in-law who created a classroom family and spent the time valuing each child for what they individually contributed to the classroom, each child felt special and that they belonged. Together, the class created a mission statement that they could live by and hold each other accountable. They had family meetings where everyone had the opportunity to share their story, including if someone was unkind to them. They learned how to communicate from how it made them feel instead of blaming and shaming someone. She was not leading the family; she guided them and encouraged them to find solutions and strategies. There is a big difference when you are told to do something versus problem solving together. As a teacher, she was working within the policies, but her goal was to be proactive rather than reactive. If the school leadership focuses on creating an environment within the school, that would do the same; it could make a significant impact on the behaviors of students.

Being an Effective Communicator: Providing the Right Information

In Chapter 11, I discussed collaboration with others and setting up a business plan. Using the collaborative approach within the school setting means that people are coming together as equals to plan and problem solve how to best help a child and create this plan. This includes the process of creating the guiding documents such as the IEP. Some people may have some increased education and insight into the child based on their background, but each person, including the parents, is an equal voice at the table. As a participant in this communication, it is important to share information based on facts and not opinions or emotions. This includes sharing the parts of a child's story that impact their experience at school. Using words that describe the positives or proactive choices for a child will be more effective than describing situations that didn't work.

Here are a few examples of statements to use:

Child's name wants to be _____ when they grow up.

They love to talk about_____

They feel most connected to a group when _____ (love language)

They respond better to _____(concrete or abstract language)

They _____(thrive/struggle) with routine.

They feel overwhelmed when _____(sensory avoiding)

They use _____to help them to get calm (calming behaviors)

The behavior you may see when they are overwhelmed is _____

The strategies that have been affective to help are _____

They also have _____going on in their life. (any other social or emotional elements)

By sharing information as clear and concise as these questions, you can effectively set a child up for greater success, as this information can then be filtered into their IEP. This information does not include their academic level or learning potential, but it will create the setting that will hopefully decrease their stressors and increase their body's readiness to learn.

If you don't know the answers to some of these questions, then you don't know enough of the story to help the child. You can gain this information through the family or caregivers or through therapy evaluations or previous teachers. This information should be shared with all those around the child so that we are all working towards unlocking this child's potential.

Being an Effective Listener and Asking the Right Questions

Being an effective listener is also very important in the school–parent relationship. Sitting in a room with all those involved in the care of a child can be overwhelming. Everyone at the table should be given their opportunity to speak. Often, there may be as many perspectives on the child's story as there are people in the room. When someone shares their opinion, we need to ensure that it is based on facts and not emotions. Is it true, and does it have facts to back it up?

Even with my own four children, I have heard stories from other people about things my children have done or said that even surprised me. Sometimes the comfort of the environment that they're in may not allow others to see certain sides of them. Remember my child who would be so overwhelmed after school? The teacher never saw that side of him, but it didn't mean it didn't exist. Therefore, there is value in hearing how a child will react in different environments from everyone at the table. Consider these clues to figuring out more about what makes a child thrive and what to avoid.

If someone around the table or someone working with a child shares information or a story about a child, it is important to ask the questions to understand what was happening to understand the whole story. If it is related to a behavior, you can ask:

> *What was happening just before the behavior occurred?*
> *What happened earlier in the day?*
> *What was the environment like? Was it loud, quiet, busy, disorganized?*
> *How did the person in charge at the time respond to the behavior?*
> *Did this make the behavior escalate or deescalate?*

Let me go back to the story I told about a boy named Carter, who struggled with anxiety and was called out by his music teacher for forgetting his instrument. He knew he forgot his instrument and was embarrassed, and his body went into a reaction that he was struggling to control. To compensate for this, he put his head down on his desk. His teacher's repeated questioning and requiring him to look up at her only aggravated the situation. She interpreted this as disrespectful. Yet, she didn't know that Carter struggled with anxiety and his behavior was how he had learned to try to self-regulate. When she spoke to the mother and learned the story, the questions about the situation made more sense to her. It comes down to perspective. We see what we have in front of us unless we understand someone's story. Understanding the why behind a behavior can open doors into how to best support and motivate a child to succeed.

Advocating for Your Child and Expecting the Best Outcome

In advocating for a child, start by believing that everyone is doing the best they can with the support and resources that they have. Understand that each person you meet will have their own story, history, experience, and expectations. As a parent, or caregiver, or advocate, always start the conversation by setting expectations and ground rules for a meeting. This can be valuable in any meeting that you are attending. Expectations are focused on what the meeting was called for and what we hope to walk out of the meeting with. It keeps everyone on track and focused. For example, if a child exhibits significant behaviors at school, a meeting for this child, which should include input from this child, would have the expectation that we are developing a plan that is going to help the child to safely and effectively develop strategies to help them continue to work towards their future vision. The focus should not just be on stopping the behavior; it should be about building the skills to navigate this and any future challenges.

By creating these expectations for the meeting, understanding how to communicate effectively, and listening, you are advocating for the child, with the expectation that we are all striving for the best outcome.

In the next chapter, I will discuss how working with health care providers can differ and how to navigate the world of specialists as it relates to a child's unfolding story.

Chapter Reflections

1. Why is it important to have open communication between home and school?
2. How can behaviors at home affect school?
3. Why can parents see behaviors at home that don't happen at school?
4. What elements of the school environment may affect a child?
5. Why is it important to provide the right information to the school?

13 Communication With Health Care Providers

When children are struggling at school or home, it can create concern for parents, caregivers, the school, and the child. To learn how to best support a child, other health care providers are often brought in to discuss the child's needs. Health care providers, such as doctors, specialists, and therapists, can significantly impact the child's unfolding storyline. Each person a child sees may have some insights into a specific area that a child may be struggling with. This will be based on their area of expertise. If you remember back in Chapter 2 when different professions were discussed, each profession has their own focus or their own lens through which they will look at a situation. This is why finding the right professional for the needs is essential. You wouldn't want to ask a car mechanic to check your vision, nor would you want your massage therapist to fix your car. You want the most qualified person in that area to answer your questions. In the same way, if you take your car to the mechanic because it is not braking very well, you would expect that they will consider all parts of the car required to brake, not just look at the brake pads.

By reading to this point in the book, you should now understand how important it is to see a child's complete story. All the pieces are intertwined into the bigger picture. It is similar to how every part of our body is connected. You can't separate the hand from the arm or the eyes from the face. Therefore, the information that we learn about one piece of the body may significantly impact another part of the body. The whole of each part's purpose and function in the body is greater than their individual properties. This means that the ear alone is not useful or valuable unless connected to the brain in order to identify the sound it receives or signal the body's sense of movement in relation to gravity.

Each system within the body also does not work in isolation. The food that we eat affects our brain and how we think, act, and feel. Moving our body can change the way we feel and help us increase our focus. Enough sleep is also required for our body to function effectively.

Think about the last time you missed a night of sleep. How did you feel the next day?

Think about how you felt sitting on the couch watching television versus going for a walk.

DOI: 10.4324/9781003166405-13

If we know the whole body interacts together to function effectively, how can we create this unity between all the professions to understand one profession's impact on another. How do we align the information so that it works together in the best interest of the child? It comes down to understanding and communication.

A very common evaluation of a child's ability to function at school is through a psycho-educational assessment. This assessment is often performed by a psychologist. One child I was working with struggles with bright lights and noises. It is in this environment that he has difficulty focusing, staying on task, and controlling his behavior. He was referred to do some testing to determine where he struggles. The challenge is that this testing takes place in a small room or office with only one person present. The room is quiet and calm. What this psychologist saw and experienced in this evaluation was a child who was able to stay focused and engaged. What was not in the evaluation was the fact that there was an absence of all the sensory triggers that overwhelm him. In essence, this was the best environment for his learning, but it is the most unrealistic in the school environment. The results from this evaluation did not fully detail how the environment might change the results. So, if the school focuses on the results of the test, without considering the environment, it is not taking into account the whole picture.

We need to remember that no specialist or health care provider has a magic key that can unlock the mysteries of a child, but they may have some insight into strategies to help understand a child and how to work towards their vision. So, how do you find the right person, and how do we communicate with this person?

Finding the Right Provider for a Child's Needs

To know what help a child needs, we must first identify what area a child is struggling with. Children may not understand how they are struggling because they don't know how other people are experiencing the world. If you have ever needed glasses in the past, you may not have realized that you were seeing blurry images or what clear vision was, until the optometrist put the lenses in front of your eyes that gave you clear vision. We can't ask a child why they didn't tell us sooner about something they are experiencing because they may not know what life is like without it. For example, a child with anxiety about taking tests may assume that everyone gets that way when they take a test. We don't know the difference until we learn the difference.

So, if a child is feeling overwhelmed and you are unsure what the concerns are or if there are global concerns, meaning in multiple areas, an assessment that looks at all aspects of a child can narrow down the focus. An example would be in occupational therapy, where the evaluation is broader and contains multiple parts that help understand the child's abilities regarding the skills required for learning. A psychologist will often also do a global assessment, referred to as a psycho-educational assessment as described earlier. This testing is to determine the academic and cognitive challenges that a child may have. If more specific needs are identified, a referral would often be recommended to someone specializing in that area. If you are seeking information off the World Wide Web, ensure that the information is coming from reputable sources such as universities, hospitals, and health organizations.

Not all specialists have the same abilities. It is essential when trying to find the right provider to understand what they offer. For example, if a child is struggling in class with following instructions, it would be recommended for the child to get their hearing checked to make sure that they are able to receive the sound. All audiologists are trained to test hearing, but not all audiologists would do the test for central auditory processing. The difference is that one will ensure that they can hear in both ears, which is important, but if they are having difficulties comprehending language, you would want to make sure that the audiologist can also assess how the brain receives the information.

This is where the referral or recommendation for a child to see a provider needs to contain the information that is pertinent to the child. When a provider understands why they are seeing the child, they often focus their attention towards the areas the child is struggling in.

In my initial assessments as an occupational therapist, I always assess a child's ability to visually recognize and see objects and words both near and far. If I notice a discrepancy, I recommend that the parents or caregivers take the child to see an optometrist to rule out any vision concerns. If a parent takes a child for a regular eye exam, it may come back as normal vision. Over the years, I have learned that it is very important for the optometrist to know some of your child's story: for example, sharing about the child's struggles, especially as they relate to the visual system. If a child struggles with reading, getting very exhausted by the end of the day, rubbing their eyes, and irritable, there may be more going on with the child's vision than just their ability to focus. A child may have 20/20 vision, which is considered normal, but may struggle with the eyes focusing at different rates, known as binocular vision, and that difference in time can make a big impact. It can be significant when children are trying to read or maintain their focus on their school work. If the muscles need to work extra hard to focus, they will be exhausted at the end of the day, which may make the child irritable. Do you see how the information made a difference to what the optometrist looked for when testing?

Navigating the world of specialists can be challenging for all those involved with a child's care, from researching which specialist is right for your child to getting a referral and then waiting for an appointment. In some places, referrals can take months to years, which can feel too long in the timeline of a child's life.

To see some of the specialized providers, there is often a referral process either from the school or through a family doctor. The information passed from one party to another may or may not include important information that can affect how a provider assesses a child. Communication is so important and can come down to mere words that can make a world of difference.

In developing my therapy business, I reached out to government officials about connecting to discuss the feasibility of partnering with them in some countrywide opportunities. They agreed to meet with me in person and had set up a meeting for the following week. They said the meeting would be downtown and asked if I could make it. I live quite far from downtown Toronto, our closest major city, but I was heading there for an appointment with my son. I thought if they could meet me close to the same time, I could arrange someone to watch my son. The meeting was confirmed, and the address was given, which was on Queen Street. I prepared for the meeting, gathered all my resources, and was ready to meet with them. When the day came, my son and I headed downtown. I even coordinated to have my father-in-law, who works downtown, meet me close to my meeting, so he could have lunch with my son and I could go alone. When the time came, I couldn't find the exact address and began to panic. Queen Street is a large street in Toronto, so I walked up and down, but all I could find at that address was a restaurant, and I knew I was meeting at an office on the third floor.

When I called to ask them to clarify the directions, she said it was close to the river. Now Toronto is not on a river, but on a lake, so I was confused. When I asked her what city she was in, she said Ottawa. For those who don't know Canada, Ottawa is five hours from Toronto and is another major city. It also has a downtown and a Queen Street. What fascinated me is that we never once clarified in what city we would be meeting in all the conversations leading up to the meeting. It was one word that made a world of difference.

This example emphasizes that clear communication is vital when it comes to information needed. One word can make an enormous difference in the outcome of a situation. Even letters can make a difference. If a child was referred for therapy or to a hearing clinic because they were hyposensitive to noises versus hypersensitive, the treatment expectations would differ—hypo meaning not sensitive to noises and hyper meaning oversensitive to noises.

Have you had a conversation with someone, only to discover you were discussing two different topics?

This has happened in occupational therapy, as we are often referred to as OTs. In the school board, OT is also the short form for occasional teacher. When I would meet with a teacher or be in the staff room during lunch and tell them I was an OT, they would start talking to me like I was an occasional teacher asking questions about the class I was covering, not realizing I was a therapist.

If I had introduced myself as an occupational therapist, the teacher would have known my background. Because I wasn't clear, it led to the confusion. Similarly, the clarity in our conversations is vital to finding the right practitioners for a child. Sharing information that is valuable can change the relationship of those they meet. So how do we communicate with health care practitioners or referral sources to understand the child's story and what the concerns are in the most effective way? What is the necessary and essential information?

Providing the Right Information

The relationship that each provider will have with the child is often very different from that of a teacher. A teacher spends most of the day with a student throughout an entire school year. They often see the child in multiple situations, such as with peers, during tests, physical education, and learning new materials. In most instances, a specialist spends only a very short time with a child. Other than a few specialists who complete a full assessment that may take a few hours, for many, it only takes a few minutes. Some therapists may also provide treatment and will spend more time with a child, but this is still short compared to the time spent at school and home. On average, an occupational therapist may see a child once per week or once every two to three weeks. Even the time that an occupational therapist spends with a child will not be enough to make a significant impact on its own. The information we learn about a child and recommendations for a child need to be incorporated into the bigger picture.

Therefore, it is the collaboration between the health care providers and the parents and teachers that will make the most impact for a student. It is also valuable to get feedback and information from the teacher, parent, or guardian. Their understanding and experience with a child will be different from what a provider will see or experience. For recommendations that are coming from the school or parent to the health care provider, the referral information needs to be clear and the right information provided.

Jamie was the mom of a daughter named Savannah. Savannah struggled at school, had difficulty focusing, exhibited outwardly aggressive behaviors towards teachers, and had difficulty sleeping. She was always in trouble at school, and no matter what the teachers tried, it would still become a fight. She was known in the school as one of the behavioral kids. The challenge was that nobody would ever see past her behaviors to understand what truly made her who she was. Her frequent visits to the principal's office forced her parents to reach out to their family doctor for help.

The family doctor recommended that a psychologist see her for a psychoeducational evaluation. This evaluation showed that Savannah was very strong in many academic areas. She did have trouble with attention and focus, and it was noticed that she had difficulty with rules, as they would make her feel that she needed to resist, which often put her in the fight mode. This evaluation was comprehensive, and they spent quite a bit of time with the child. From what was found in the assessment, the psychologist determined that Savannah would benefit from seeing a psychiatrist in regard to the medication recommended to help her with some of her diagnoses.

Throughout this, Jamie had always mentioned that her daughter behaved differently when she slept better, but part of her issue was that she had difficulties getting to sleep at night. The psychologist said that the psychiatrist would be the best person to talk about that. When Jamie went to the psychiatrist with Savannah, the challenge was that the psychiatrist already had the report from the psychologist, which gave him all the information that he thought he needed. From this report, he recommended a specific type of medication and left no time to get more of the parent's story.

After starting the course of drugs, one of the side effects was that it would also affect sleep. It created more problems for Savannah in terms of her fatigue, not being able to settle, and it affected the rest of the family's ability to sleep. When Jamie tried to reach out to the doctor, his concern was more on the medication and if it was effective for helping Savannah with her focus and attention. There is a lot more to medicine and weighing the risk and benefits that we are not focused on in this book, as this can be complex. The purpose of this story is that the mother's concern was more on the frustration of not getting across how much they were struggling at home with the lack of sleep.

Like other parents, this caused Jamie to look into helping her child sleep better by approaching other professionals. Savannah had sleep studies and went to see a naturopath, homeopath, and massage therapist. The struggle was that none of these were effective because of the side effect of the medicine, which Savannah was still taking.

The mom became frustrated because she was trying to piece all the issues together without fully knowing how they interacted with each other. She felt like no one was listening to her and that no one was helping her get to the source of the issues with her daughter.

So, how can a parent communicate with professionals so that they can understand what the provider is thinking and also feel that they expressed the right information to the professional concerning their child? How do you effectively provide this information?

Start with ensuring that all those involved with the child are focused on the same concerns.

Child's name is working towards becoming a _____
They are very strong at _____ skills
They are having difficulties with _____
   (specific struggles)
This is affecting them by _____ (behavior that is
   displayed)
They thrive in _____ environment
They struggle in _____ environment
We are looking for strategies to _____ (goal
   from visit)

This is why it is valuable to set expectations for an appointment. Creating a document like this and expressing goals keeps everyone focused on the concerns. This can even be sent in a short letter to the provider before a first visit. It will give the provider a chance to review the information before an appointment and understand the concerns. If the provider can't offer answers on strategies or recommendations, they may be able to recommend the next steps for the child.

When I work with parents, I often have them create a more complex document that includes all the information that they have learned about their child, as outlined in this book. These questions were highlighted in the last chapter for consideration when communicating with the school. The parents can highlight their child's sensory needs, love language, learning needs, the behaviors that their child will display when they are overwhelmed, and what it looks like when they are trying to self-regulate. The goal is to empower parents with the knowledge and words to explain their child to others involved in their care. When you empower someone with knowledge, it increases their confidence in making changes and being involved in the care. It is never a finalized document; it is a working document that will change over time. What it has created is a way to share a child's unfolding story with others.

Being an Effective Listener and Asking the Right Questions

Each health care provider is there to help navigate and provide strategies to help a child. The information they provide based on their perspectives or lens should be geared to the child's best options at that moment. The communication from each provider in regard to a child should be given at a level that all of the people involved can understand. In the same way, rationale and options need to be outlined clearly to those involved. It is about informing, especially those responsible for the child, about all aspects pertaining to a recommendation.

In our story earlier, Savannah was started on a medication to help her with her focus and attention. The specialist who recommended that medication should have been clear on why he chose that medication and outlined both the risks and benefits and alternate options. It would have allowed her mom to make an informed decision knowing the other options that exist. Having this open discussion creates a more collaborative approach because it will enable people to understand their options and have some say in the decision. Part of the discussion should have also been on the risk and benefits of the medication's side effects regarding sleep. Treating one aspect of a child's life and not looking at how it will affect the rest of the person is similar to treating the foot separate from the leg.

Part of the treatment rationale from providers needs to consider the capacity of the parent or caregiver. Many treatment recommendations involve the cooperation and collaboration of those involved with the child. If this is not within their current ability, then alternate options need to be concerned.

Likewise, if there is a financial requirement for a recommendation, we need to be aware of the family's financial abilities. It may be the best option for the child, but it may not be reasonable or financially feasible. We then need to inform them of all the options so that the parent/caregiver can make their own decision. This may include providing information and resources for services that can help them financially.

Health care providers need to understand and evaluate each person individually, as each person's and family's story will be different. The information that providers give to parents also needs to be clear and concise. I recommend to parents or guardians that they receive rationale behind any treatment decision to understand each decision's breadth and depth. If a provider is not clear in their communication, I have highlighted some key questions a provider could be asked to ensure that information is communicated clearly to answer what a parent hopes to hear from a provider:

Based on the findings _____ from our discussion,

I recommend_____

This the best option because_____

The side effects or risks include _____

Alternate options would be _____

They are different because _____

This will affect the child in the future by _____

Is this a reasonable option?

Are there any questions?

Health care providers also need to remember that they may not be the only person involved in this child's care. If a parent has gone to an optometrist who has recommended vision therapy, then went to a psychologist who recommends group therapy, and the physiotherapist recommends one-on-one therapy sessions, this may be a lot for the parents to decide what is best for their child. How does another treatment fit into this, and what takes priority over another if a parent has to choose? Within all the options, we need to make sure that each person contributing is effectively working towards the same goals for the child.

In navigating the world of health care providers, I have heard parents refer to it like a job on its own, and they can find appointments disruptive to children who thrive on structure and routine. Parents also say that their children act differently with the providers, and it is not an accurate picture of what everyday life is like. With my children, having different appointments for the four of them is nearly impossible to schedule. When a specialist only sees a snapshot of a child's life, they may not fully grasp the entire picture. It really does take some time to truly understand a child and all that makes up a child and how they navigate and react to different situations.

Advocating for a Child and Expecting the Best Outcome

In advocating for a child, just like discussing a child at school in Chapter 12, start by believing that everyone is doing what they think is best for the child. They are doing this from their professional perspective or lens. Yet, we need to remember that every person whom a child meets or works with is still human and has their own story, history, experience, and expectations.

As a parent, or caregiver, or advocate, always start any conversation with a specialist by setting expectations for a meeting as we discussed earlier. Even if the meeting is with one specialist, it ensures the expectations are focused on what the meeting was called for and what information we hope to know when we leave the meeting. It keeps everyone on track and focused. By creating these expectations for the meeting, understanding how to communicate effectively, and listening, you are advocating for the child, with the expectation that we are all striving for the best outcome. For example, if you book an appointment for a child's vision and you want to know about their binocular vision, make sure to include that when you are booking, in case it requires more time. Then once a child is in the appointment, start the conversation by stating why you are there. Explain the challenges your child is experiencing and what you hope to discover.

When advocating, you want to make sure that all the information received is clear, and if it is not, return to the questions in the previous section on how to listen effectively. Never assume that someone understands the child or views the child in the same way. Clearly communicate what the child's story is so that everyone is working from the same information. The choices made for a child when they are young can significantly impact their future. We need to remember not to get stuck in this moment and get through tomorrow; we are helping them build the skills that will help them navigate their future.

It brings us back to the discussion in Chapter 11 on creating a vision for a child. By setting the vision, each time we meet with different professionals and advocate for a child, we need to ensure that we are still working towards that vision. Do the recommendations align with the child's mission, or does it have negative impacts? If the recommendation for a child is to go to group therapy to work on behavioral skills, but the child is not comfortable in groups, it may cause more anxiety and stress than good. It may be better to choose another available option that does not increase the anxiety and stress as a starting point.

Then, within the vision, you have long-term goals and short-term goals. If the short-term goals are to add medication to help a child like Savannah, what is the long-term goal? Understand how this plan is going to be monitored and what the intention of this choice of treatment is.

Remember that no one has a magic pill that changes the way a child acts, thinks, or learns. If someone is offering this, run far away. In most cases, each person working with children is passionate about the knowledge and insights they have learned about their area of expertise and how it can help a child. The goals should be aligned with the child's needs and meeting the child where they are—not trying to meet the world's needs around them. Navigating all of the specialists and health care providers can feel overwhelming for everyone. With the number of people who have a different perspective on the child, you need to make sure that they are taking into account the whole person and ensure that their recommendations align with the overall vision. Each child is unique, and we should be helping them to reach their greatest potential.

Chapter Reflection

1. What is different about working with health care providers than with the school?
2. Why is it important to find the right provider for a child's needs?
3. Why is it important to be clear in our communication?
4. Why is it valuable to set expectations for a meeting upfront?
5. Why is it important to advocate and expect the best outcome?

14 Conclusion

The information I covered in this book is only the starting point of all the different aspects of a child. The goal of this book is to help everyone around a child to understand that there is more to a child than what we see on the outside. It is about changing our focus and modifying the way we see the world. Instead of seeing only the flower's petals for its color and beauty, by changing the focus, we can see what else the flower needs to survive. We can see the soil that is holding the roots, the stem that is transporting the water, the leaves that are processing the sunlight, and we can see the environment that it is growing in. It is hard to take our eyes off the colors of the flower, but that part of the flower wouldn't exist without the other parts, and each flower is unique and beautiful. Children are like flowers. We see the outward appearance, yet there are so many parts that need to work together for the child to reach their greatest potential. The most important is a supportive environment that will make the flower flourish.

Working with children is one of the most rewarding yet challenging professions. It is amazing to watch a child learn and explore the world. Yet, when something is bothering them, it can be hard as parents, therapists, and caregivers to figure out exactly what or why something is creating that experience for them. This is where it can feel challenging. It often takes patience and curiosity to spend the time discovering a child's story and what makes them who they are.

When you start to understand parts of a child's story, you can see the beauty within them. You can see how a child can light up the world. Understanding and communicating a child's story takes time, but it will have exponential returns, and as a child continues to grow and develop, so does their story. They begin to learn more about themselves and the world around them, just as we did while we were growing up.

As you have read through this book, I hope that you have recognized that you have your own story as well. We each do. It is not just for children. It is our unrepeatable story. Meaning no one's life will ever be the same as ours, and this our one story. Even writing this book, I realized how many events and memories have changed the trajectory of my life. Good or not-so-good experiences alike have made us who we are. We can't change the past, but we can

DOI: 10.4324/9781003166405-14

learn from it, and we can create a better future. Every story is a story worth telling.

Remember the Beginning

If you are reading this and trying to think about where you can start going through this process with a child, start at the beginning.

Remember that a child wouldn't exist if it weren't for the people who created them. The first step is to understand who is raising the child and what their story is. Much of a child's world is influenced by the environment they are growing up in. Often, when we are looking at a child, we forget that they are the product of other beings. It includes their genetic makeup, which includes some factors that children are predisposed to. Understanding this can give us valuable information. A child brought up in different cultures, ethnicities, and economic statuses may have different views and experiences of the world. What a child or caregiver has seen or experienced may be beyond our imagination. We cannot assume that all children are raised in the same manner. Therefore, it is vital to start with understanding who is raising the child.

When we understand who the caregivers are, we need to check in with them if we notice something has changed with a child. This is the first place we should touch base, as we know that having changes at home can impact a child outside of the home. I worked with a child who was always energetic and happy for therapy sessions. During one of our sessions, I noticed that she was super quiet and not really engaged. After a few minutes of working together, she said she was really sad today. Her grandmother had passed away. She was not close with her grandmother, but she said it made her sad because her mom was really sad and had been crying all night. Sometimes, although children may not understand all that goes on in the adult's world, they can feel the stress, anxiety, and sadness. I changed our therapy session that day to find joy and happiness and give her some space. We made a card for her mom, giving the child a way to feel like she was doing something to help her mom not be so sad.

We need to recognize that big or small events can affect a child each day. They are human beings just like us, and it is important to check in with the child or the parents to find out if something has changed.

Think About What Makes a Child Unique

Each child is unique in how they look, act, and experience the world. Their reactions will continue to change as a child grows and develops; both their body and abilities will change.

Start by recognizing and acknowledging a child's physical differences, as this will give us key information. We need to go beyond looking at physical differences or physical disabilities and focus on a child's abilities. A child lacking fingers may be a fantastic artist, as a child lacking legs may be a fast runner.

When we focus on a child's abilities, we change the focus from what they can't do to what they can accomplish. It is like giving a child wings and watching them fly. Often children given the proper support and conditions can do amazing things. Think about Nic Vujicic, who was born without arms or legs. Many would doubt his capabilities as a child, but he is inspiring people all around the world by his abilities.[8]

Each step beyond this point delves deeper and deeper into discovering how a child experiences the world through their senses. Watch how a child engages in their environment. Listen to stories from those around them, and ask questions about when the child is the happiest and most engaged. Then do the same, including observing to see trends of when a child disengages or misbehaves. Ensure that you activate all of your senses in the discovery, including what we touch, see, taste, smell, hear, and the way we move about the world. to understand our body's position against gravity or our body's relation to itself. We also need to know how aware a child is to their body's own ability to signal when they need to go to the washroom or when they are hungry. The information you collect from all your observations will be key information to set up the right environment that includes eliminating stressors, creating a calming space, and giving clues to understand their behaviors.

By going through the process described earlier, while you watch and engage with a child, you can recognize how a child processes information. Remember that children hear and understand the information in different ways. The same sentence may take on very different meanings to other children. Even the directions such as clean your room can take on different meanings. Even amongst my four children, I get four different results. We often forget about the words we use and the definitions they may have. We forget that what we know may not be understood by others. To some, it may sound like we are speaking a foreign language. Try different ways of saying the same command and observe the difference. See how many steps or instructions a child can remember. What you will learn from this can affect a child's school environment and how they engage in class and classwork.

Similarly, how children retain information is relative to what a child has experienced or understands. I notice this the most when I work with young children learning how to print. The formation of the alphabet letters is not innate and needs to be taught for kids to learn it. Children would often do better with letters if they were related to games or activities they knew. The letter "*e*" *starts by hitting the baseball and running the bases. The letter "j" is like the hook on a fishing rod. The letter "i"* looks like a candle. We learn best when we can connect to anchors in our brain from pre-existing knowledge.

Similarly, children may struggle with writing a story about a horse, but will be able to write a whole page on dinosaurs. The stronger the links in our brain, the easier it is for us to find the information to create a story, which is also true when it comes to motivation to learn. If you were told you needed to learn how a lawnmower works, but you have no interest in this topic, you will not be interested or motivated to learn. If we can connect value and meaning to the purpose, we can increase motivation. If a child is frustrated in learning, connect them to a topic of interest and see if it changes their abilities.

As children continue to grow and change, we need to continuously re-evaluate all these factors to see how they have changed and how it impacts a child's engagement.

Set Up the Environment for Success

Once you have the information about their sensory and learning needs, the next step is to set up the environment to meet their needs. The environment can significantly impact how a child engages based on all the information you collected. Like we reviewed in this book, the environment is more complex than just the physical space, but the physical space is a good place to start. Setting up the physical space to be conducive to a child's needs and creating accommodations or modifications when necessary can set a child up for success.

Allowing a child to put on headphones in a noisy room during work time may be enough to allow a child to find a sense of calm in an otherwise loud environment. Creating a space in their bedroom or at the back of the classroom for a child to go to if they feel overwhelmed will help them relax their body and mind. Allowing a child to play with fidgets or chew gum in class can increase their focus and allow them that release of extra energy. These are only examples, but they highlight that, sometimes, the changes are only small, but when you know what they are targeted at, they can make a significant difference.

In the same way, be aware of the social environment and how a child connects with others. How do they relate to others at home? Recognize the other children in the room. What needs do they have? How does the child relate to the teacher, support staff, or principal? A child who is being bullied by a classmate may engage differently when that child is present than when that child is away. A child may fear the principal, which may keep their behavior in check, only to have their behavior explode as soon as they leave school. It is the people a child associates with who can impact their feeling of belonging. In this book, we discussed a child's love language—understanding that we may receive love from others in very different ways. Receiving love impacts our sense of belonging, which is an innate need for all human beings.[11] If a child feels most loved when someone says kind words about them, yet at school the teacher doesn't want to highlight individual children, this may cause a child to feel that they don't belong. To feel valued for who you are and to be able to be your authentic self should not only be encouraged, but it should be expected to make this world a better place.

Imagine a world that is judgment free and recognizes and values people's uniqueness. Oh, what a world that would be!

What the Behaviors Are Trying to Tell Us

When behaviors do arise, and they often do, think of them more like the warning mechanism telling us that something isn't right. In a children's movie, this was once depicted as little warning lights going off inside our brain. When we can understand how children experience the world through their senses and how they learn, it takes on a new perspective of how and why they behave. Behaviors are an outward display of an internal struggle. It can often be confused by others as purposeful actions, and if we respond to what we see, we are not focused on the cause of the actions. Instead, we should use these displays as signs that we may need to re-evaluate how the child is processing the environment. Has something changed? What was the trigger? Did something happen at home?

Remember that behaviors can result from various stressors. The key is to figure out the stressors, try to eliminate or separate from the stressors, and then learn how to calm our bodies in relation to the stressors.[20] A child may get angry at a parent or teacher when asked to do an activity or task. Yet, if we focus on the idea that every child would do well if they could, we can change our mindset to believe that there is something about the activity or task that the child feels they do not have the ability to complete. It may not be the entire task; it could even be the sense of overwhelm of where to begin. To ask a child to write a story can seem like a big task to them, but you could start with the task of picking a topic, which is the first step to writing a story. The second step would be to brainstorm some ideas for the topic, and the third step would be to put them into sentences. This difference in instructions can make a significant change for a child who is feeling overwhelmed. What if we went a step further and instead of having so much focus on writing, we incorporated oral storytelling as an activity? How would children's reactions or engagement differ?

The mistaken beliefs of children also play into how they behave. Children will subconsciously believe stories about how they can achieve their sense of belonging. Remember that it is our innate desire to feel a sense of belonging and significance.[9] Be inquisitive when a child is misbehaving and see what they might be trying to tell you. Even ask. A child may share their feelings, and it may be different from your assumptions.

Believe in a child's capabilities. If we encourage and allow children to participate and engage in life, they will also believe in their capabilities, increasing their feeling of value and belonging.

The Balanced State

In all the information you have collected or noticed, the key is to figure out how to get a child to learn to return to a balanced state. This can be very challenging for children, who often need guidance until they can learn how to achieve this balance independently. The term for finding the balanced state is self-regulation. Think about when you are upset or angry. What do you do to find your sense of calm? Often, as adults, we walk away, take some time for ourselves, do some deep breathing, have a cup of tea, or journal. All these strategies allow our body and mind to return to balance. Finding what works for children is more challenging, as often what works for us will be different. Even what works for one child may be different from others.

As a child grows and changes, what worked last month, last week, and today may be different. What is more important is that they understand what that feeling is when they feel balanced, and you can help them find ways to get there.

Helping children learn how to self-regulate will be different in different environments, but this skill will help them navigate a world that we can't control.

Communicating the Story

Discovering a child's story is one step, but sharing it is another important step. After you have collected all the information, you need to share it. Finding a way to communicate a child's needs with others in a way that is well received may impact how a child functions in different environments. Remember that this is not the language that everyone speaks, so ensure that you share their needs in a positive and proactive way. The goal is to focus on who the child is and what the future holds and not what they have done. Remember the importance of setting a vision and goals for a child beyond today and beyond this moment. Our vision for a child should be focused on reaching their greatest potential, not for them to be a better-behaved student.

Knowing a child's story is especially important for parents to understand and recognize their child's needs. Often, they are the child's best advocate, and they should feel empowered knowing their child's story well enough to share it with others. This knowledge empowers parents to be able to communicate the child's story and needs to the various providers that the child works with.

All the key features or characteristics that we have discovered about the child need to be included in the child's story, including their abilities, sensitivities, calming strategies, behavioral reactions, and learning styles.

We are all unique and have a different unfolding story that even once you share it, you need to keep revisiting and rewriting it.

This book is intended to be a starting point for understanding a child's potential. We often focus on one aspect of a child, such as their behavior, lack of focus, or physical limitations, and we miss some of the other important parts that make them unique. When working with children, start at the beginning, be curious, and recognize what makes them who they are. Remember that there is a story behind every child and every person. No child is the same, and no two stories are the same. Each child deserves to have their whole story told. We should not only help each child, but also believe in the ability for a child to reach their greatest potential.

Acknowledgments

This book was a culmination of passion and purpose. My belief is that often-misunderstood stories needed to be shared so that others would not be misunderstood. Years of life and work experience gave me the insight to put these words together. Thank you to all the families that allowed me to be a part of their child's journey over the years.

This book was also written in an unprecedented time in history, as we were faced with a global pandemic, with many parents, including myself, having to guide children through academic, emotional, and social changes. All of these demands highlighted the importance of recognizing each person's unique story and how each was experiencing the world.

I want to especially thank Karen Graham for her guidance and support through the intricacies of writing this book and seeing not only the forest, but also "the bark in the forest." I would not have been able to see this through without her.

Thank you to Hilary, Robin, Trang, and Catherine, for your belief and support throughout this process and continuous motivation that this book was worth writing. Thank you to all those I met on my entrepreneurship journey who encouraged me to follow my passion and believed in my potential from the Accelerator Centre, Rhyze Ventures, and Laurier WEC. Thank you to friends near and far who supported me through my career and this endeavor in various ways.

Thank you to the editors at Routledge Publishing who believed in my vision for this book and your willingness to share this vision with the world.

Thank you to my supportive parents who through your actions always taught me that I could achieve anything I set my mind to. To my amazing sister and friend: you inspired me to be an occupational therapist while I watched your career as an occupational therapist impact so many lives. You have been my mentor in so many ways. To all my other family members and in-laws, thank you for always supporting my endeavors.

Thank you to my husband who has supported me through all my dreams and encouraged me to follow my passions.

Finally, but not least, thank you to my children, who have taught me so much about life and about how wonderfully and beautifully each one of us is made.

Thank you for teaching me how to be a better mom and person. Spending this last year unexpectedly endeavoring in the adventures of homeschooling you has been one of the best years of my life. I am excited to continue to watch each of your stories unfold and support you to reach your greatest potential.

I hope this book inspires each person out there to look at life through a lens of curiosity and believe in each person's potential.

Bibliography

1. Shaw, G. (2020, June 29). A scientific study claims that your age affects how you see this famous optical illusion. *Insider*. www.insider.com/study-says-age-affects-optical-illusion-2018-9
2. Knowles, F. E., III. (1995). Memories of Dr. Dunton. *Maryland Psychiatrist Newsletter*, *22*(3) (para. 3). www.dunton.org/archive/biographies/William_Rush_Dunton_Jr.htm
3. Canadian Association of Occupational Therapists. (2016). *Who we are and what we do* (History section). https://caot.ca/site/wwa/whoweare?nav=sidebar
4. Townsend, E. A., & Polatajko, H. J. (2007). *Enabling occupation II: Advancing an occupational therapy vision for health, well-being, & justice through occupation.* CAOT Publications ACE.
5. Law, M., Cooper, B. A., Strong, S., Stewart, D., Rigby, P., & Letts, L. (1996). The person-environment-occupation model: A transactive approach to occupational performance. *Canadian Journal of Occupational Therapy*, *63*, 9–23. doi:10.1177/000841749606300103
6. Tsabury, S. (2010). *The conscious parent: Transforming ourselves, empowering our children* (p. 22). Namaste Publishing.
7. Dweck, C. S. (2016). *Mindset: The new psychology of success* (p. 6). Random House.
8. Vujicic, N. (2010). *Life without limits* (Kindle ed.). Crown Publishing Group.
9. Nelsen, J. (2006). *Positive discipline* (Kindle ed.). Random House Publishing Group.
10. Brown, B. (2010). *The gifts of imperfection* (p. 26). Hazelden Publishing.
11. Chapman, G., & Campbell, R. (2016). *The five love languages of children*. Northfield Publishing.
12. Biel, L., & Peske, N. (2018). *Raising a sensory smart child*. Penguin Random House.
13. Pfaffmann, C. (2017, February 17). *Human sensory reception*. Encyclopædia Britannica. www.britannica.com/science/human-sensory-reception
14. Shaywitz, S. (2003). *Overcoming dyslexia*. Vintage Books.
15. Bodison, S., Watling, R., Miller Kuhaneck, H., & Henry, D. (2008). *Frequently asked questions about Ayres Sensory Integration®*. American Occupational Therapy Association. www.aota.org/-/media/Corporate/Files/Practice/Children/Resources/FAQs/SI%20Fact%20Sheet%202.pdf
16. Riener, D., & Willingham, D. (2010). The myth of learning styles. *Change: The Magazine of Higher Learning*, *42*, 32–35. https://doi.org/10.1080/00091383.2010.503139

17. Oakley, B., Sejnowski, T., & McConville, A. (2018). *Learning how to learn: How to succeed in school without spending all your time studying; A guide for kids and teens.* TarcherPerigee; Illustrated edition.

18. Chbosky, S., Conrad, S., Thorne, J., & Palacio, R. J. (Screenplay). (2017). *Wonder.* [Movie]. Lionsgate, Participant Media, Walden Media, TIK Films, and Mandeville Films

19. Greene, R. W. (2014). *Lost at school.* Scribner.

20. Shanker, S. (2017). *Self-reg: How to help your child (and you) break the stress cycle and successfully engage with life.* Penguin Canada.

21. Dreikurs, R., & Stolz, V. (1991). *Children: The challenge: The classic work on improving parent-child relations* (Reissue ed.). Plume.

22. Greene, R. W. (2014). *The explosive child: A new approach for understanding and parenting easily frustrated, chronically inflexible children* (5th rev. ed., Kindle ed.). Amazon.ca

23. Williams, M. S., & Shellenberger, S. (1996). *How does your engine run?® A leader's guide to the Alert Program® for self-regulation.* Albuquerque, NM: TherapyWorks, Inc. www.thealertprogram.com

24. Kuypers, L. (2021). *Zones of regulation: Framework designed to foster self-regulation and emotional control.* www.zonesofregulation.com/index.html

25. Hanscom, A. J. (2016). *Balanced and barefoot: How unrestricted outdoor play makes for strong, confident, and capable children.* New Harbinger Publications.

26. Ramsey, D. (2011.) *EntreLeadership: 20 years of practical business wisdom from the trenches* (p. 31). Howard Books.

27. Google. (n.d.). *Our approach to search* (para. 3). Retrieved February 17, 2021, from www.google.com/search/howsearchworks/mission/#:~:text=Our%20company%20mission%20is%20to,a%20wide%20variety%20of%20sources.

28. Nike. (n.d.). *What is Nike's mission?* (para. 1–2). Retrieved February 17, 2021, from www.nike.com/help/a/nikeinc-mission

29. Covey, S. (2015). *The 7 habits of highly effective people.* Mango Publishing Group.

Continued Reading

Chapter 1

Shaw, G. (2020, June 29). A scientific study claims that your age affects how you see this famous optical illusion. *Insider*. www.insider.com/study-says-age-affects-optical-illusion-2018-9

Chapter 2

Townsend, E. A., & Polatajko, H. J. (2007). *Enabling occupation II: Advancing an occupational therapy vision for health, well-being, & justice through occupation.* CAOT Publications ACE.

Chapter 3

Dweck, C. S. (2016). *Mindset: The new psychology of success.* Random House.
Townsend & Polatajko, 2007.
Tsabury, S. (2010). *The conscious parent: Transforming ourselves, empowering our children.* Namaste Publishing

Chapter 4

Brown, B. (2010). *The gifts of imperfection.* Hazelden Publishing.
Chapman, G., & Campbell, R. (2016). *The five love languages of children.* Northfield Publishing.
Nelsen, J. (2006). *Positive discipline* (Kindle ed.). Random House Publishing Group.
Vujicic, N. (2010). *Life without limits* (Kindle ed.). Crown Publishing Group.

Chapter 5

Biel, L., & Peske, N. (2018). *Raising a sensory smart child.* Penguin Random House.
Kranowitz, C. S. (2006). *The out-of-sync child: Recognizing and coping with sensory processing disorder.* Penguin Publishing Group.
Kurcinka, M. S. (2015). *Raising your spirited child, third edition: A guide for parents whose child is more intense, sensitive, perceptive, persistent, and energetic.* Harper Collins.
Shaywitz, S. (2003). *Overcoming dyslexia.* Vintage Books.

Chapter 6

Dweck, 2016.

Greene, R. W. (2014). *Lost at school.* Scribner.

Oakley, B., Sejnowski, T., & McConville, A. (2018). *Learning how to learn: How to succeed in school without spending all your time studying; A guide for kids and teens.* TarcherPerigee; Illustrated edition.

Chapter 7

Dreikurs, R., & Stolz, V. (1991). *Children: The challenge: The classic work on improving parent-child relations* (Reissue ed.). Plume.

Greene, 2014, *Lost at school.*

Greene, R. W. (2014). *The explosive child: A new approach for understanding and parenting easily frustrated, chronically inflexible children* (5th rev. ed., Kindle ed.). Amazon.ca

Nelsen, 2006.

Chapter 8

Biel & Peske, 2018.

Greene, 2014. *The explosive child.*

Kuypers, L. (2021). *Zones of regulation: Framework designed to foster self-regulation and emotional control.* www.zonesofregulation.com/index.html

Nelsen, 2006.

Williams, M. S., & Shellenberger, S. (1996). *How does your engine run?® A leader's guide to the Alert Program® for self-regulation.* TherapyWorks, Inc. www.thealertprogram.com

Shanker, S. (2017). *Self-reg: How to help your child (and you) break the stress cycle and successfully engage with life.* Penguin Canada.

Siegel, D. J., & Bryson, T. P. (2012). *The whole-brain child: 12 revolutionary strategies to nurture your child's developing mind.* Bantam Books.

Chapter 9

Hanscom, A. J. (2016). *Balanced and barefoot: How unrestricted outdoor play makes for strong, confident, and capable children.* New Harbinger Publications.

Chapter 10

Greene, 2014, *The explosive child.*

Nelsen, 2006.

Shanker, 2017.

Chapter 11

Covey, S. (2015). *The 7 habits of highly effective people.* Mango Publishing Group.

Ramsey, D. (2011). *EntreLeadership: 20 years of practical business wisdom from the trenches.* Howard Books.

Chapter 12

Biel & Peske, 2018.
Greene, 2014, *Lost at school*.
Nelsen, 2006.
Shanker, 2017.

Author Biography

Sabrina E. Adair, MScOT, is a practicing occupational therapist and a passionate advocate for parent empowerment. She is a mom of four beautiful children who have taught her patience, perseverance, and compassion and that we're all wonderfully unique individuals with our own unfolding stories. Sabrina's experience working with children has inspired her drive for innovation and inter-professional collaboration. In 2019, she founded Enabling Adaptations, a private therapy company focused on helping parents and caregivers to find ways to effectively understand and communicate their child's needs in order to create positive environments where children can reach their greatest potential. Sabrina is an award-winning entrepreneur and shares her successful approach to improving children's lives at speaking engagements, parenting workshops, and more. Sabrina holds a post-professional Master of Science in Occupational Therapy from Dalhousie University and a Bachelor of Science in Occupational Therapy from the State University of New York at Buffalo. Sabrina resides just outside Toronto, Ontario, with her husband and children.

Index